caring for people with dementia

Sara Miller McCune founded SAGE Publishing in 1965 to support the dissemination of usable knowledge and educate a global community. SAGE publishes more than 1000 journals and over 800 new books each year, spanning a wide range of subject areas. Our growing selection of library products includes archives, data, case studies and video. SAGE remains majority owned by our founder and after her lifetime will become owned by a charitable trust that secures the company's continued independence.

Los Angeles | London | New Delhi | Singapore | Washington DC | Melbourne

caring for people with dementia

a shared approach

Christine Brown Wilson

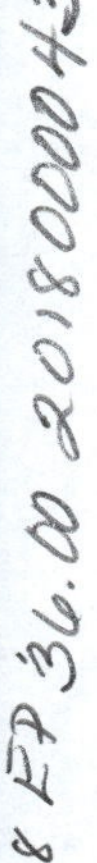

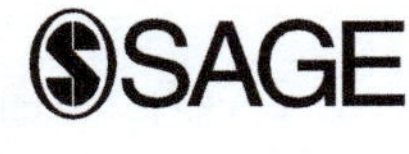

Los Angeles | London | New Delhi
Singapore | Washington DC | Melbourne

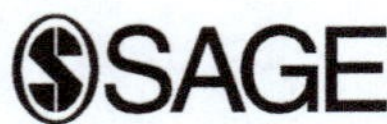

Los Angeles | London | New Delhi
Singapore | Washington DC | Melbourne

SAGE Publications Ltd
1 Oliver's Yard
55 City Road
London EC1Y 1SP

SAGE Publications Inc.
2455 Teller Road
Thousand Oaks, California 91320

SAGE Publications India Pvt Ltd
B 1/I 1 Mohan Cooperative Industrial Area
Mathura Road
New Delhi 110 044

SAGE Publications Asia-Pacific Pte Ltd
3 Church Street
#10-04 Samsung Hub
Singapore 049483

Editor: Becky Taylor
Assistant editor: Charlène Burin
Production editor: Katie Forsythe
Copyeditor: Jill Birch
Proofreader: Thea Watson
Indexer: Gary Kirby
Marketing manager: Tamara Navaratnam
Cover design: Wendy Scott
Typeset by: C&M Digitals (P) Ltd, Chennai, India
Printed and bound by
CPI Group (UK) Ltd, Croydon, CR0 4YY

First published 2017

Library of Congress Control Number: 2016954243

British Library Cataloguing in Publication data

A catalogue record for this book is available from the British Library

ISBN 978-1-4129-6199-8
ISBN 978-1-4129-6200-1 (pbk)

Contents

About the author

Christine is an Associate Professor at the University of Queensland, Australia currently holding the position of Director of Teaching and Learning in the School of Nursing, Midwifery and Social Work. Prior to this Christine was a Senior Lecturer at the University of Manchester in the UK, where she worked with a number of organisations interested in improving dementia care. Christine's research is interdisciplinary as she works with social workers, psychologists and engineers to consider novel solutions to real world practice problems. Christine adopts a partnership model of research involving people with dementia, family caregivers and staff. Whilst in Manchester, Christine led a Care Homes Research Interest Group that brought together academics, care organisations, healthcare staff, people with dementia, family caregivers and direct care staff to determine the questions that needed to be asked in research proposals.

Christine's research focuses on relationship-based approaches to care and how to improve the experience of people with dementia, their families and staff. Since returning to Australia, Christine has been working with indigenous organisations to explore the cultural transferability of relationship-based approaches to care. Christine is also working with family caregivers and people living with dementia in the community to consider how families and communities may provide support and further resources in living well with dementia.

Christine has published widely in academic journals and her first book, *Caring for Older People: A Shared Approach*, was published by Sage in 2013 with positive reviews. *Caring for Older People: A Shared Approach* explains in depth how to apply relationship-based approaches to care in a range of settings drawing on the perspective of older people, families, staff and students. This book: *Caring For People With Dementia: A Shared Approach*, applies the same principles within the context of organisations, demonstrating how we can all make a difference when caring for people with dementia by working together at every level of the organisation.

Foreword

This book is about enabling person-centred and relationship-centred care in practice and highlights the importance of culture in advancing this perspective. Dr Brown Wilson calls this perspective relationship-based approaches to care. An important message she shares in the introduction of the text is: 'To achieve the best care possible, we need to prepare nurses and other health care practitioners with the skills and attitudes to provide effective culturally responsive care'. As a dementia researcher and health professional I am very supportive of this statement and I would like to promote this book as one way to help readers and students to prepare for the practice of evidence-based care of people with dementia. Dr Brown Wilson's message encouraged me to reflect on several situations in my teaching, research and family where relationship-based approaches to care were espoused but often not connected within practice. I share some of these reflections below in the hope that they demonstrate the importance of culture and relationship-based approaches to care.

Some years ago when I was teaching a postgraduate class about dementia I was confronted half way through the semester by a small group of students from a culture outside of Australia. These students argued with me that they didn't know why I was teaching subjects such as person-centred care, relationship-centred care and non-pharmacological approaches to care as these practices went against what was accepted and current practice in their country. For example, in their culture if a person with dementia was agitated or aggressive the family or health professional would manage the person and situation by giving them psychotropic medication and tying the person to a chair or locking them in a room. They argued that this resulted in the problem being contained: there was no longer a problem for staff or family of an agitated or aggressive person, and this was acceptable in their practice. I felt the floor opening up to me as I realised my teaching was representing an Australian culture of care and I had neglected to allow students the opportunity to examine their beliefs and practices in relation to evidence-based relationship approaches to care. This was a perfect opportunity for me to reflect on my teaching practice and to consider alternative ways to assist students from any culture to discuss and to understand why some practices even though they are common are not best for the individual. I hope readers of this text will also be open to practices that may be new to them and to take note of the approaches outlined by Dr Brown Wilson in this text.

A few years ago when asking staff from a residential aged care facility to tell me about their philosophy of care they all quickly expressed that the philosophy of care in their organisation was person-centred care (PCC). However, not one of these staff could tell me what they did in their practice to advance PCC. They knew the words but they didn't know how to play out such a philosophy within the care situation, as

PCC was not incorporated or truly embraced within their organisation. Unfortunately even today I continue to see similar examples where PCC sits in broad statements within an organisational mission statement but is not truly practised. This text will help readers to understand the importance of culture and the impact of culture on care provision.

Furthermore, we know that health and care staff are told not to get too close to patients/residents, as this will implicate their care. Therefore everything must be conducted at an arms distance so that staff don't get involved with the individual as this can also emotionally implicate their situation. As a result we find communication is more likely to take place between staff to staff and limited communication takes place between staff and an older person with dementia. It is very challenging to provide a relationship-based approach to care if we do not 'know' the person and yet so often the culture and policies within an organisation can prevent this happening.

Finally, I would like to reflect on a positive care approach that was presented to one of my family members. The staff in this situation understood PCC and the importance of relationship-based approaches. Unfortunately like many readers of this book, my family too has been touched by dementia with two grandfathers, a father, and sister-in-law all receiving a diagnosis of dementia. My grandfathers both died while being given little respect or dignity in the care they received. The care was far from a relationship-based approach to care. The approach was one that ignored the person while concentrating on the tasks at hand. In recent years I found my father's situation was quite the opposite of what I had witnessed previously. My father ignored his dementia diagnosis and continued to teach in his swimming school a squad of young people who were in my father's eyes future champions. They accepted his memory problems and his sometimes erratic behaviour as they trusted and admired his strengths. He had formed a strong bond and closeness to the students over the many years he had taught them. Several months before the passing of my father he spent a horrible two months in an acute care hospital for a comorbid condition. He became angry and aggressive toward staff and his condition deteriorated significantly to the point where he was no longer able to return home. He was very agitated on admission to a nursing home and we talked at length about his impression of the facility and staff. He didn't want to be there and as the facility was not secure he talked of walking out of the door to go home. Staff were given an extensive personal history and his prominence in the community meant that several staff had crossed paths with my father as a result of his long running business. Unbeknown to me staff told a 'white lie' – by informing him that the facility once a week took the residents to the local physiotherapy pool (true for a small group) and they would like to offer him the role of volunteer swimming coach for the residents. They brought a white board into his room and my father used the board to write training programmes for the residents. He was at last focused on something he knew and had spent his life developing. I smiled as he confessed to me that he was working hard on the training programmes, however he was concerned that some of the residents were old and he didn't know if they would be up to his rigorous schedules. He was heartened that others saw his potential. This activity gave him back his dignity, staff and residents enjoyed talking with him about the training programmes and in his eyes he was once again an important member of society. I hope that readers can also see this as a fine example of staff being truly involved in patient care and with a focus on the person's strengths.

Furthermore, this book aims to help readers (students) to lead and manage change through the organisation as a Complex Adaptive System and relationship approaches to care. I am in awe of Dr Brown Wilson for this aim as too many authors focus only on PCC and ignore the important perspective of relationships, culture and partnerships in care. I trust that readers of this book will move into practice with a focus on the integration of relationship approaches in the care they provide. I also hope that they will be better equipped to navigate the challenges of the complexities of organisations that care for older people. It is imperative that an ageing population has advocates that can make positive changes to practice. Importantly I hope readers and teachers will benefit from the numerous activities offered in each chapter of this text and the opportunity to reflect on their reading.

Professor Wendy Moyle
Menzies Health Institute Queensland
and School of Nursing and Midwifery,
Griffith University, Brisbane, Australia

Acknowledgements

This book would not be possible without the people who live daily with dementia, their family caregivers and the organisations that support them who have given generously of their time to speak with me over the past ten years. I am indebted for the many stories shared with me that have been instrumental in demonstrating how multiple and shared perspectives underlie relationship-based approaches to care.

I have been privileged to work with and alongside a number of people living well with dementia dealing with the everyday challenges the condition brings. In particular I would like to thank Peter Ashley for his expertise with the SensorMat project and Dr Ann Johnson for her support with research and teaching at the University of Manchester. I have also had the privilege of speaking alongside Christine Bryden in Australia. Thank you all very much for your time and energies and the inspiration provided by your life experience.

It has also been my privilege to work with organisations that truly make a difference in the lives of people with dementia. Working with Community Integrated Care (C-I-C) in their development of the Each Step Dementia model demonstrated how an organisation could integrate relationship-based approaches to care at each level of the organisation. This experience forms the foundation of this book and I would like to thank Michelle Phillips, Manager of Each Step and the Executive Team for their support during my consultancy with C-I-C.

There have also been colleagues upon whose experience I have drawn heavily, in particular, Professor Ruth Anderson and Associate Professor Kirsten Corrazini in their work on Complex Adaptive Systems in the USA and also Professor Marilyn Rantz and her team at Tiger Place in Missouri who are developing innovative technologies. In Australia, I would like to thank Professors Wendy Moyle, Nancy Pachana and Elizabeth Beattie for both their welcome and invaluable support as I returned back to Australia.

This book would not have been possible without the support of the publishing team at Sage: Becky Taylor, Emma Milman, Charlène Burin and Katie Forsythe. Thank you for your patient support as you saw the many deadlines come and go. I also need to thank my great friends Jane and Rob for their very generous hospitality at their Blue Mountain retreat, without which, this book may never have been started. Although last, never least, are thanks to the tireless support of my husband Terry and daughter, Amee and son, Leigh as I juggle and chase the many deadlines that seem to define academic life. Terry as always has spent many hours proofreading these chapters and Amee has used her graphic design skills in producing the figures to near impossible timeframes. Thank you all for your patience and your love.

Publisher's acknowledgements

The publishers would like to thank the following individuals for their invaluable feedback on the proposal and chapters of the book:

Donna Doherty, Staffordshire University, UK
Angela Kydd, University of the West of Scotland, UK
Fiona Lundie, University of the West of Scotland, UK
Dr Sarah J. Rhynas, University of Edinburgh, UK
Genevieve Thompson, University of Manitoba, Canada
Sally Underwood, The University of Sheffield, UK

The author and publishers are also grateful to the following for their kind permission to reproduce material:

Figure 1.1: Adapted and reproduced with kind permission from 'World Alzheimer Report 2011: The benefits of early diagnosis and intervention' Alzheimer's Disease International

Table 6.2 : Alzheimer's Society (2013). Building dementia-friendly communities: A priority for everyone. London: Alzheimer's Society.

Introduction

Dementia is a global public health issue; 46.8 million people worldwide are living with dementia and 7.7 million new cases are being diagnosed each year, the majority of which are in middle to low income countries (Prince et al., 2015). Alzheimer's disease has been the second leading cause of death since 2011 in England and Wales with a similar ranking in Australia (Australian Institute of Health and Welfare, 2012). In the USA death resulting from dementia has risen by 11–15% in 2014 (National Center for Health Statistics, 2015). The cost of dementia is either matching or exceeding other chronic conditions such as cancer, heart disease and stroke (Prince et al., 2015). The total cost of dementia to society in the UK is £26.3 billion, with an average cost of £32,250 per person (Prince et al., 2014). The impact of dementia is also felt at an individual and community level as dementia is a condition which shortens people's lives and affects quality of life of the individual as well as family and friends (Prince et al., 2015). As the ageing population increases, the amount of people living with dementia will also increase, particularly in the over-85 age group, who represent the fastest growing proportion of the population.

Dementia is a progressive syndrome affecting the brain resulting in deterioration of memory, thinking, and the ability to undertake everyday activities. Dementia is a result of underlying disease, of which Alzheimer's disease is the most common. Everyone is affected differently by dementia, nonetheless dementia does impact on a person's ability to reason, make judgements and recognise everyday objects (World Health Organisation, 2015).

There is no cure for dementia but promising breakthroughs have been made in gene therapy to restore damaged brain cells (Tuszynski et al., 2015) and also in the application of ultrasound to remove the plaque associated with Alzheimer's disease (Leinenga and Götz, 2015). Whilst research into a cure continues, the focus is now moving towards prevention as with other chronic conditions. The 'Nun Study' (Snowdon, 1997) demonstrated that many people could live with the pathology of Alzheimer's disease without developing dementia. Cohort studies from around the world have subsequently demonstrated that people with healthy lifestyles are less likely to develop dementia. Barnes and Yaffe (2011) in reviewing the risk factors associated with dementia determined that with lifestyle modification, there was the potential to reduce the incidence of dementia by 10–25% if all seven risk factors were reduced (see Figure I.1). The message now is that we need to maintain a healthy brain to improve cognitive reserves and so reduce either getting dementia or have the brain in a healthier state to manage the dementia.

Reduce
saturated fats
Balanced diet
No smoking
Moderate
alcohol intake
Reduce
blood pressure
Prevent diabetes
Physical &
leisure activities
Cognitive
stimulation

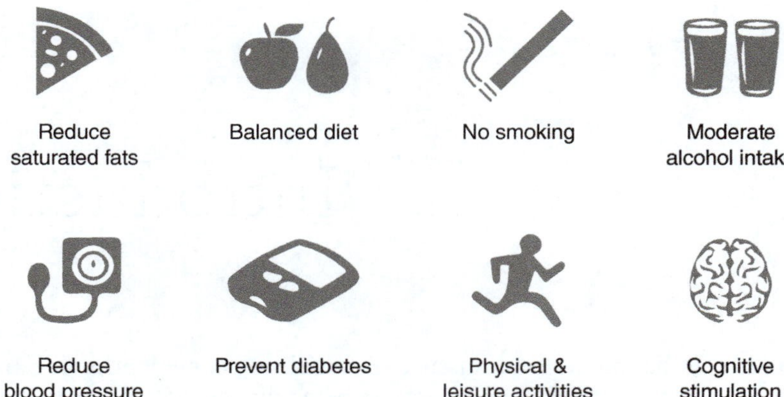

Figure I.1 Reducing our risks

As we have seen from the initial prevalence figures, the rate of people developing dementia is increasing, particularly in the oldest old age groups, which means that there will be more people requiring care and support as they age with dementia. Care, therefore is becoming an overriding concern for all governments as the rate of people being diagnosed with dementia increases (WHO, 2015). This situation is further complicated by migration. Many people are ageing in countries to which they migrated as younger people and now form communities of culturally and linguistically diverse (CALD) populations within these host countries. These communities are often in minority groups and so are likely to have more adverse health outcomes when compared to the majority of the population. Many countries with a colonial past will also have indigenous communities in places such as Australia, Canada and the United States. A further cultural group is the Lesbian, Gay, Bisexual, Transgender and Intersex (LGBTI) population whose needs are often under-recognised in cultures that are predominantly heterosexual. Many LGBTI peoples experience discrimination and marginalisation similar to other minority cultural groups (National LGBTI Health Alliance, 2014). Therefore, we need to ensure we have responsive services that meet the needs of people with dementia and their families from culturally diverse backgrounds. To achieve the best care possible, we need to prepare nurses and other healthcare practitioners with the skills and attitudes to provide effective culturally responsive care.

Culture itself is a dynamic rather than a static concept and everyone belongs to cultural groups with a common set of beliefs and attitudes that bring them together. Cultural awareness is being aware that we see the world through our own individual cultural lens. Cultural sensitivity means we acknowledge that other cultural groups see the world differently, accepting that there may be variation between the beliefs of diverse cultural groups and our own. Cultural competence is developing a set of skills and behaviours that enable us to work effectively with culturally diverse and indigenous communities. However, competence implies a final position being reached whereas cultural responsiveness is a process of self-reflection and learning that supports the healthcare practitioner to proactively respond to the changing needs of the person, family or community with whom they interact (Indigenous Allied Health Australia, 2015). Culturally responsive care could be considered an extension of person-centred care, paying particular attention to social and cultural factors in managing therapeutic encounters with patients from different cultural and social backgrounds (Carteret, 2010). Throughout this book, cultural responsiveness remains an implicit principle beneath the philosophies of person-centred and relationship-centred care. Adopting a biographical approach to care planning is the starting point to find out what matters to people but further work may be needed to create communities in which all people feel valued for their culture and/or sexuality.

Person-centred care (PCC) is well established as a philosophy of care and has a developing evidence base across a range of environments that provide care and support for people living with dementia. However, it is evident from the many poor reports about the experience of people with dementia and their families that PCC remains challenging to realise in day-to-day care. There is also limited research when considering how PCC transfers across cultures that have a more collective or community focus. Relationship-centred care (RCC) (Tresolini et al., 1994) was developed with a community focus and has been applied to a range of healthcare environments (Nolan et al., 2001; Ryan et al., 2008) although there has been limited work to consider how RCC translates across cultures. This book integrates the perspective of person-centred and relationship-centred care within an organisational framework to support the reader in exploring what is needed at each level of the organisation to ensure that direct care reflects person-centred or relationship-centred care. Examining how different strategies might work at the different levels of the organisation will empower students to manage change in their individual practice in the short term with a view to being equipped to lead and manage change following graduation. Equally, this book is relevant to postgraduate students and those in positions of management who wish to make a sustainable difference to the care being delivered for people with dementia in the organisation in which they practice.

Dementia is a journey; the experience of this journey has implications for the person with dementia, their families and staff in the services providing support. The practice scenarios throughout this book draw on the perspective of people living with dementia, family caregivers and staff in a range of environments to demonstrate how PCC and RCC can be implemented in practice so that we, as healthcare practitioners, can support the journey being made. This means the focus is often on everyday care routines and how people work together in teams to deliver care since a critical mass of staff with a similar motivation is needed to deliver consistent care across shifts (Brown Wilson, 2012). The approach to care will be influenced by the organisation in which care is delivered and this book adopts the perspective of organisations as Complex Adaptive Systems (CAS) as the mechanism to support organisations in achieving the vision of person-centred and relationship-centred care. Adopting the lens of CAS provides a series of practical strategies at each level of the organisation to support person-centred and relationship-centred care in everyday routines founded on partnership working with people with dementia, families, communities and staff.

This book is designed to do two things: firstly to introduce students to partnership working with people experiencing dementia, families, communities and other staff; secondly to focus on how practice might need to change to ensure people with dementia receive the best outcomes.

Pre-registration students remain supernumerary in practice in the UK and many countries influenced by the UK system such as Australia and Singapore. In the UK, supernumerary status remains a requirement of the Nursing and Midwifery Council for the preparation of nurses, ensuring they enter the workforce fit to practice. This supernumerary status enables students to undertake personal care routines where relationships are built and individual stories shared. Students are rarely supported to understand the importance of these stories or how to use them to positively influence the care of people with dementia. The value of storytelling in collecting biographical information is highlighted as a crucial starting point for the development of person-centred and relationship-centred care. Storytelling is often an accepted medium within CALD and indigenous communities for the sharing of relevant information and is an approach that can be beneficially incorporated into healthcare systems when supporting people with dementia. Articulating how biography can be used in care planning is the initial step in developing PCC and contributes to the development of shared understandings that underpin RCC. Practice scenarios and activities throughout this book provide the stimulus for students to critically examine the application of practical strategies at different levels of the organisation. We start with a person-centred focus (*micro*), followed by considering how the needs of the person, the family members, staff and others within the community might be met using a relationship focus (*meso*), connecting these micro and meso levels with what is required in the wider organisation (*macro*) to maintain PCC and RCC.

This book uniquely offers an organisational framework to examine the facilitators and barriers in the practical implementation of person-centred and relationship-centred care, so providing an adaptable framework for dementia care. An adaptable framework for implementing dementia care enables students and staff to work flexibly adapting to the relevant focus, whether they work in specialist or general care environments. The scope of this book includes a broad range of caregiving issues that impact the experience of the person with dementia, their families, communities and staff in providing and experiencing care. For a more in-depth discussion on specific clinical or caregiving issues readers are encouraged to look at the many excellent and in-depth textbooks on dementia care – see as an example, *Excellence in Dementia Care* (second edition) edited by Murna Downs and Barabra Bowers (2014).

Reports of people living with dementia receiving poor care has to become a thing of the past. Nurses and other healthcare professionals need to be equipped with skills that enable them to lead and role model good practice in dementia care and this book provides students with evidence-based practical strategies that have been implemented in practice environments. How these strategies make a difference to the experience of people with dementia, their families and staff is clearly explained. This book is designed to be easy to read, leading the reader along a pathway with clear signposts, encouraging the reader to consider the evidence base and develop practical strategies thus enabling them to implement PCC and RCC in practice. The organisation of the book supports critical thinking in relation to both theory and practice demonstrating how the reader can achieve collaborative working including people with dementia, their families and communities. All readers will be challenged to consider how they might influence organisations to ensure high quality care that improves the experience for people living with dementia, families and staff.

Chapter 1: Common myths associated with the condition known as dementia

Common societal myths frame this chapter to take the reader through the dementia journey. The current evidence is examined to challenge the common myths about dementia encouraging the reader to focus on the person with dementia's experience of this journey. An overview of the trajectory of dementia is provided from assessment to end of life with relevant reference to international perspectives in dementia care. Best practice from different countries is presented to support people with dementia, their families and communities throughout their journey. Evaluating what is meant by best practice provides the reader with a useful starting point for considering the relationship-based philosophies in Chapter 2.

Chapter 2: Developing relationship-based approaches to dementia care

Dementia care is all about relationships; therefore this chapter focuses on the different philosophies of dementia care that promote the value of relationships. The principles and evidence for individualised, person-centred and relationship-centred care are examined alongside activities that promote a critical evaluation of how these approaches might be implemented. This chapter contends that relationship-based approaches to care occur along a continuum and following this discussion, the term relationship-based approaches to care (Brown Wilson, 2012) will be used as shorthand for individualised, person-centred or relationship-centred care in the remainder of the book.

Chapter 3: The role of the organisation in leading and facilitating relationship-based dementia care

Considering organisations as Complex Adaptive Systems rather than hierarchical systems is examined as a lens through which we might view organisations when implementing relationship-based approaches to care. This chapter considers the theoretical perspective of Complex Adaptive Systems and the leadership required to facilitate relationship-based approaches to care. A range of practice scenarios based on the literature and the author's practice development experience encourage readers to consider how everybody in the organisation might develop positive relationships, influencing relationship-based approaches to dementia care.

Chapter 4: Developing a biographical approach in care practice

Recognising the personhood of the person with dementia is a fundamental principle of all relationship-based philosophies. Seeing the person begins with a biographical approach to care planning where we value the stories people with dementia, families and communities share. This chapter will examine barriers and enablers at the care delivery or the micro level of the organisation when using a biographical approach to care planning that might impede or promote relationship-based approaches to care. The reader will be taken through the process of developing biographical knowledge in completing a care plan that adopts a relationship-based model of dementia care.

Chapter 5: Managing relationship-based approaches to care

Person-centred care may often be dependent upon the staff currently on duty. Alternatively, staff may perceive positive achievements with people with dementia as 'lucky' rather than attributing such achievements to a relationship-centred strategy. This chapter encourages the reader to articulate strategies that promote relationship-based approaches to care and how they might be developed using a team approach. Leadership at the meso level of organisations is explored to develop a consistent approach for people with dementia and their families. The reader is encouraged to complete a development plan thus enabling them to implement relationship-based approaches to dementia care.

Chapter 6: Creating dementia-friendly services

Many businesses aspire to providing a dementia-friendly service but it is not always clear if organisations that espouse a person-centred philosophy actually deliver this in practice. Organisational culture and how this influences policies and the physical environment will be explored. This chapter encourages readers to engage with the macro level of an organisation in order to identify how the organisation might facilitate relationship-based approaches to dementia care. By the end of this chapter, the reader will have revised policies and developed an organisational plan to implement a dementia-friendly environment.

Chapter 7: Developing community through dementia-friendly environments

Returning to the micro level of the organisation, this chapter considers the personal and social environment for the person with dementia. Many people with dementia experience Behavioural and Psychological Symptoms of Dementia (BPSD). What this means for the person, the family and staff is examined. Different approaches to understanding the meaning and supporting behaviour of the person with dementia are explored. This chapter concludes with a consideration of how an organisation might implement education and training ensuring staff are equipped to support people with dementia in their practice.

Chapter 8: Supporting the families of people living with dementia

Family caregivers are vital in supporting people with dementia. Family has many meanings across different cultures and readers will be encouraged to examine how partnership working can be implemented within the culture of communities in which they work. The meaning of relationships in the wider family will be explored and a range of interventions aimed at supporting family caregivers critically evaluated. Activities will support the reader in developing a partnership working plan for families they are supporting.

Chapter 9: The role of technology in dementia care

Technology is constantly being developed for dementia care from the use of surveillance and GPS monitoring to robots in providing care and/or emotional support. As this technology becomes embedded in everyday life, its use in formal dementia care will inevitably rise. This chapter examines the current debates in the types of technology being developed and how this might impact on implementing relationship-based approaches to care. Strategies to involve the person with dementia, families and staff in the development and implementation of technology are explored, culminating in a framework to involve people with dementia and their families in decisions involving technology.

Chapter 10: Leading and managing change in dementia care

To embed relationship-based approaches to care, leadership and the management of change will be necessary. This chapter examines how relationship-based approaches to care influence quality outcomes for the person with dementia, families and staff. Readers are taken through a step-by-step process in a single Quality Improvement methodology to implement relationship-centred approaches to care taking into account each level of the organisation.

Conclusion: Making a difference

This conclusion returns to the metaphor of a journey to summarise the key messages in the implementation of relationship-based approaches to care. A journey is not the same as a holiday that can be pre-planned and is often time limited. A journey may take a person down unexpected pathways that can be either supportive or challenging. Everyone's journey may be different but by the end of the journey, many people will be changed by their experience. The role of professional services when supporting people with dementia and their caregivers is to provide support as they journey, recognising that each person's journey will be unique to them. This final chapter returns to the continuum of care, locating how leadership, working in teams and partnership working enables organisations to move along the continuum to person-centred and relationship-centred care.

I hope you find this book both challenging and stimulating as together we implement relationship-based approaches to dementia care.

1

Common myths associated with the condition known as dementia

Learning objectives

By the end of this chapter, the reader will be able to:

- Identify common myths and stereotypes associated with dementia.
- Critically discuss relevant evidence to dispel common myths and stereotypes relating to people with dementia.
- Explain the trajectory of dementia from assessment to end of life.
- Reflect on the implications for practice when working with people living with dementia and their caregivers.

Introduction

Dementia is a misunderstood term associated with a range of myths and stereotypes. This is due to many people not being aware what is meant by the term or why dementia might affect different people in different ways. The purpose of this chapter is to thoughtfully examine some of the myths around dementia that give rise to stereotypes, which may influence our thinking and our practice. To begin, let us examine why we need to consider dementia as a separate issue within our practice.

Dementia is a global phenomenon with over 46 million people affected worldwide. It is anticipated that 9.9 million cases of dementia will be diagnosed globally each year representing a global cost of US$818 billion (Prince et al., 2015). Dementia impacts on the individual, the family and wider society with caregivers of people with dementia providing more care than other disabling conditions such as stroke (Prince et al., 2015). Dementia is not a result of the normal ageing process but there is a greater likelihood of more people experiencing dementia as the population ages (Australian Institute of Health and Welfare, 2012; ADI & WHO, 2012). However, it is not older people alone that are at risk of dementia as there exists an increasing cohort of younger people receiving a diagnosis of 'Young Onset Dementia'. Therefore, with growing numbers of people across the lifespan likely to experience dementia, this condition is now being recognised as a public health priority at a global level (World Health Organisation (WHO), 2015). This means that in whatever context you practice, you will need to be equipped with the skills, attitudes and knowledge to care effectively and safely for people living with dementia. This chapter aims to examine and dispel some of the common myths associated with dementia. The myths are arranged to represent the journey that people living with dementia and their caregivers may well follow. This will provide you as a nursing and healthcare professional with a deeper insight into what people living with dementia and their caregivers might have experienced in the time before they required the service you are working within. This will provide you with an opportunity to examine the implications for your practice when working with people living with dementia and their caregivers.

What is dementia?

Dementia is a progressive syndrome that causes deterioration in a person's memory, language, personality, behaviour and ability to perform everyday functions. Dementia itself is not the disease process but rather the impact of the disease process on the person. Dementia is described as an umbrella term representing symptoms that might emerge from over 100 conditions such as Alzheimer's disease, vascular disease, Frontotemporal Dementia (FTD), Korsakoff's Syndrome and Lewey Body's (Alzheimer's Australia, 2015). The symptoms that affected individuals display depend on the underlying disease process and where it affects the brain. For example, FTD often affects a person's personality leading to behaviour change where the family identify this as not representing the person they once knew. Sexual disinhibition is also related to FTD.

Different types of dementia may also affect language and the ability to understand what is seen or heard, creating difficulties in communication. Progression of dementia is variable and differs according to the underlying condition and person. Irrespective of when people begin to exhibit signs or receive a diagnosis the progression of dementia along with signs and symptoms may vary from person to person. This can be challenging for professionals, families and those in the community alike as everyone has a mental image of what it is to have dementia. For many dementia has negative connotations of losing one's mind or not being able to care for oneself. Holding these negative images of dementia may result in many people rejecting the notion that you could live a positive life with dementia.

Diagnosis is an important part of the dementia journey and in effect signals the start of the journey. Whilst diagnostic labels are of benefit in the classification and treatment of disease, they may also bring stigma and stereotyping (Garand et al., 2009). Stigma has been described in Goffman's seminal work as setting people apart, and labelling them as 'the other'; this then moves on to stereotyping all people with the same label as having the same attributes and then giving society permission to treat 'them' differently (Goffman, 1963). This situation is evident in people being diagnosed with dementia as society withdraws contact from those who may not fit the societal norms of behaviour, hygiene or dress (Graham, 2003). As the dementia progresses, the person living with dementia finds it increasingly difficult to process multiple signals within social situations and respond according to social expectations. As a result, the person with dementia may receive negative reactions from others, resulting in additional stress for both the person and their caregivers. Subsequently the decision may be taken to not go out or meet up with friends, resulting in isolation of the person with dementia and their family caregivers (Garand et al., 2009).

Activity 1.1 Reflection

- Identify a situation where a person with dementia was admitted to the organisation in which you were working or on placement.
- What did the staff say about this person? Was the language positive or negative?
- What were the attitudes being expressed? Were these about what was happening or what might happen?
- Were these attitudes based on knowledge of this person or on stereotypes derived from past experiences?
- How did this influence the care the person received?

The reflective activity above is designed for you to consider how our attitudes and language influence our practice. When we are working in busy healthcare environments with competing and complex demands, nurses in particular tend to see the person with dementia as taking up more time than is available. This is often because the person with dementia is in an unfamiliar environment with their usual routines now disrupted. We will return to this experience in subsequent chapters to identify how this situation might be changed at both an individual practice and institutional level.

Poor practice often arises when healthcare staff operate on myths and stereotypes rather than considering the experience of the person for whom they are caring. Equally, people living with the early signs of dementia and their family caregivers may also subscribe to the same societal myths. For these reasons, we as healthcare professionals need to remain aware of the range of myths that may inhibit people from accessing early diagnosis or additional support as the dementia progresses. There is no single set of common myths relating to dementia. However, the following section identifies many of the common myths that relate specifically to the person with dementia's journey from pre-diagnosis through to death. These are designed to provide an overview for the healthcare professional as a precursor to providing person-centred care and creating dementia-friendly environments where the person with dementia and their caregiver is respected and valued.

The first three myths focus on the person with dementia's perspective in context to the different time points of diagnosis. Understanding these issues from the perspective of the person receiving the diagnosis of dementia will support us as healthcare professionals in understanding the journey many people have been on before they are in regular receipt of services. The remainder of the myths reflect the perspective of professionals, and sometimes family caregivers, as the dementia progresses. These are the myths that often stand in the way of person-centred care.

Myth 1: 'Memory loss is a normal part of ageing and doesn't mean I have dementia'

The cognitive changes that occur as part of the normal ageing process are primarily related to additional time required by the older person in processing and/or responding to information. It may take longer for the connections to be made, but the connections can still be made. However, the issues related to memory loss in dementia are due to the connections being lost within the brain. This may be due to vascular changes (such as occlusions from vascular changes in the brain) or the formation of amyloid plaques and tau tangles that have now been associated with Alzheimer's disease. Prince et al. (2011) have developed four time periods that follow the trajectory of dementia when diagnoses might be possible (Figure 1.1). However, recent advances in brain research have changed current thinking in what represents an 'early diagnosis' of dementia (Brooker et al., 2014). For example, it is known that the plaques and tangles in the brain that have been associated with the cognitive impairment of Alzheimer's dementia may be in the brain for many years before any symptoms emerge. This stage is referred to as a prodromal period where no clinical signs are apparent. However, there is insufficient evidence on the ability of different biomarkers to adequately calculate the risk of the person with these plaques and tangles to go on to develop dementia.

The first time point representing the earliest point of diagnosis would be the detection of neuropathology demonstrating changes in the brain with no concurrent clinical signs experienced by the person. To achieve the earliest point of diagnosis, the development of sophisticated biomarkers is required. Whilst some biomarkers have been identified this field of research is still very experimental and there is no real evidence that this time point could be established.

The second time point would be when individuals and those who know them well notice changes to the individual's abilities. Cognitive tests at this point may result in a diagnosis of Mild Cognitive Impairment (MCI) which has been described as a prodromal syndrome to dementia. Although people with MCI are at increased risk of developing dementia, there is also evidence to suggest that MCI may not always progress to dementia (Albert et al., 2011; Han et al., 2012), which in turn may create uncertainty as to what this diagnosis means (Frank et al., 2006). These early cognitive

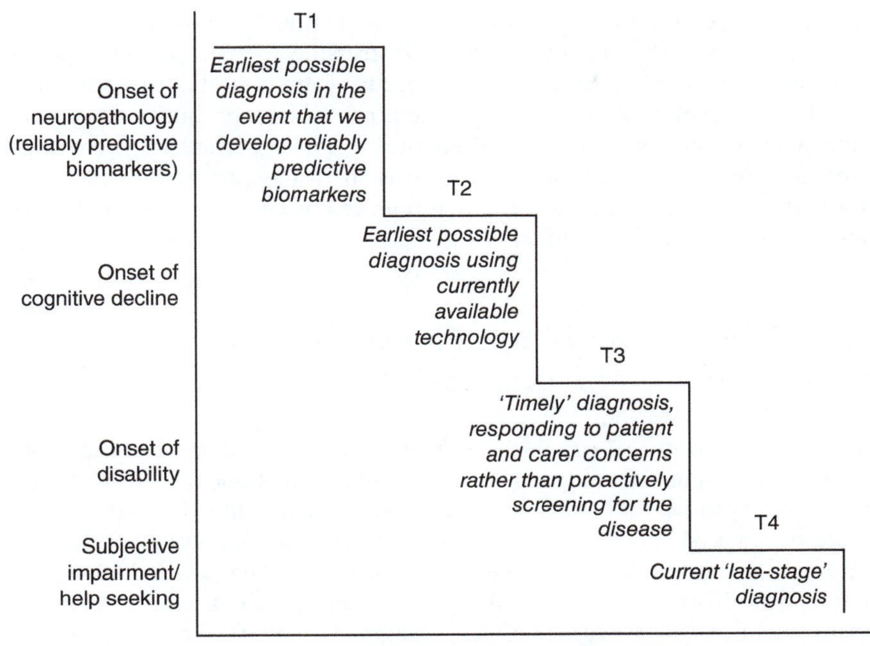

Figure 1.1 Four time points for diagnosis in the trajectory of dementia

changes may manifest in a person forgetting names, places and having difficulty with remembering recent events, difficulty in finding the right word, changes in depth perception and being easily distracted without this interfering with their daily life (Alzheimer's Society, 2015). However, those receiving a diagnosis of MCI subsequently report anxiety, fear of embarrassment, loss of skills resulting in changes in social and family roles and loss of self-confidence (Frank et al., 2006). Whilst this would be the earliest possible opportunity for diagnosis of dementia with current technology, there are also counter views that early diagnosis at this time point might be counterproductive for the person or their supporters due to the lack of pharmacological or other treatments for MCI (Brooker et al., 2014).

Activity 1.2 Reflection

- If you had a friend or relative who was behaving differently, how would you approach them?
- How would you raise any concerns you might have that it was dementia?
- Considering the person's usual routine, what factors would you consider might indicate dementia rather than forgetfulness?

We have considered the first two early time points regarding potential diagnosis for dementia. Early cognitive changes may be distressing for the person experiencing them and also for their families. These may occur over a period of time and are often described by families as knowing that something was wrong but not being able to describe what exactly was wrong. Often the person experiencing these cognitive changes may deflect concerns stating that it is their age or that they have a lot to think about. This perception may also be influenced by the next myth that even with a diagnosis nothing could be done.

Myth 2: 'There is nothing that can be done so what is the point of a diagnosis?'

Diagnosis is critical to identify what part of the brain is affected so that potential treatments both pharmacological and non-pharmacological can be explored. Diagnosis needs to be conducted by a geriatrician or psychiatrist with expertise in dementia or via a Memory Clinic to identify the type of dementia as this may provide an understanding of how symptoms progress. Diagnostic tests generally include medical history, brain imaging, physical and psychiatric assessment as well as neuropsychological assessment. Once a diagnosis is made pharmacological treatments are available for people with mild to moderate stages of dementia. The push for early diagnosis at time point 2 (Figure 1.1) is to ensure people have access to these treatments when they are likely to be most helpful. The most common type of pharmacological therapies are cholinergic drugs that block the actions of an enzyme called acetylcholinesterase which destroys an important neurotransmitter for memory called acetylcholine. These pharmacotherapies offer some relief from the symptoms of Alzheimer's disease for some people for a limited time. They are currently approved for use for people with mild to moderate Alzheimer's disease (Table 1.1). Memantine is the first in a new class of therapies currently approved for use for people with moderately-severe to severe Alzheimer's disease. Memantine targets a neurotransmitter called glutamate that is present in high levels when someone has Alzheimer's disease and acts by blocking glutamate thus preventing too much calcium moving into the brain cells causing damage. Providing a diagnosis of the type and severity of the disease enables the appropriate drug to be prescribed that will be most effective for the person thus helping them to retain function. People with dementia often say how these drugs have given them their life back and so the effect of a diagnosis should not be underestimated. Whilst these drugs do not halt the disease process, they may delay the movement between the stages of dementia or promote improved functioning even as the person proceeds through the stages of dementia.

The onset of disability that impacts on everyday functions and routines is often the point at which the individual experiencing cognitive changes or their family and friends may seek help. This is the third time point noted where a dementia diagnosis would be considered timely (Prince et al., 2011; Brooker et al., 2014). Brooker et al. (2014) suggest that help seeking initiated by the person experiencing cognitive decline and/or their family is the point at which a timely diagnosis is essential.

Table 1.1 Definitions of stages of dementia

Stage of dementia	Description
Mild	Symptoms include memory loss related to recent events, disorientation in time, difficulties with tasks requiring problem solving and reduced interest in hobbies. These symptoms might manifest in the person needing to be prompted when undertaking personal care and/or needing to be reminded about appointments. The person might not be able to recall recent events in conversation.
Moderate	Symptoms include severe memory loss with difficulties in finding words. The person finds it difficult to orientate to both time and place without support and has severe problems with judgement and problem solving. This means the person will require substantial assistance with personal care and other activities of daily living to maintain functioning in the home and the community. The person may get lost easily and begin to display behaviours such as repetitive questioning, shadowing the family caregiver, wandering, aggression and disinhibition.
Severe	Symptoms include severe memory loss including not recognising familiar people with limited language skills. The person is unable to problem solve or make judgements, requiring substantial assistance with personal care. Behaviours described as challenging for caregivers generally increase.

Depending on the person and disability being experienced, this may be at the mild or moderate stages of dementia, but for some, diagnosis may only come at the point of severe impairment. Even when help seeking is initiated, dementia may not be diagnosed due to lack of access to clinicians able to give a diagnosis or even the belief of professionals themselves that nothing can be done following a diagnosis (Prince et al., 2011; Brooker et al., 2014). As new drug therapies become increasingly available, timely diagnosis is needed to enable people with dementia and their families to gain maximum benefit from these therapies. Not everyone wishes to have a diagnosis and this should also be respected. However, once a person seeks help, then there are four sequential steps to a timely diagnosis (Figure 1.2) that should be co-ordinated at the individual/ family level as more than one professional may be involved (Brooker et al., 2014).

Brooker et al. (2014) provide comprehensive recommendations for timely diagnosis of dementia. Many of their recommendations centre on the importance of education and training for professionals in the community alongside appropriate referral pathways to ensure the correct people are involved at the earliest point. However, late-stage diagnosis (Figure 1.1) remains the norm (Prince et al., 2011; Brooker et al., 2014). Late-stage diagnosis occurs when there is significant evidence of cognitive decline on objective testing with associated disability. This may be too late to gain the benefit of treatment to enable people to remain longer within the community and may increase the difficulties experienced by families as demonstrated in Practice scenario 1.1.

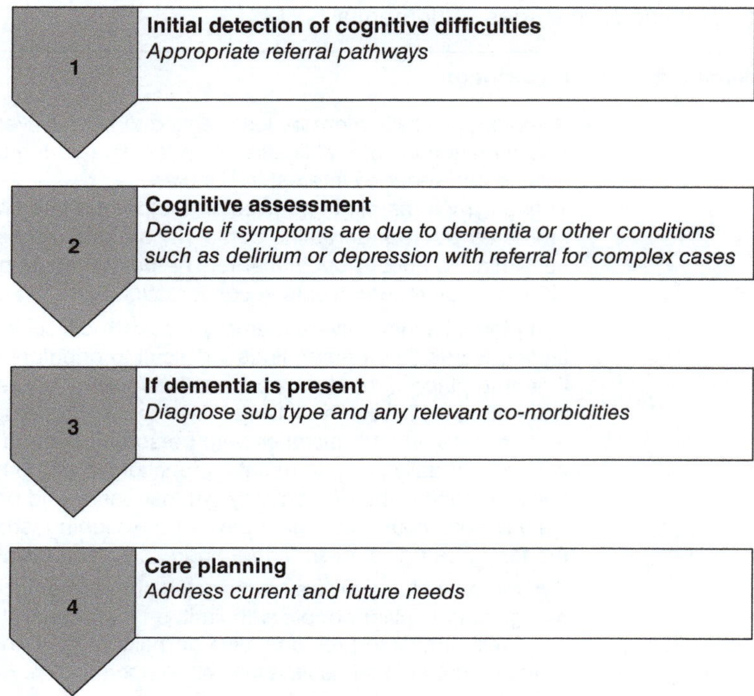

Figure 1.2 Stages of a timely diagnosis, based on Brooker et al. (2014)

Practice scenario 1.1

One daughter described her experiences of getting a diagnosis for her father as a roller coaster ride. She first noticed her father was having difficulties when she was visiting one weekend and her father thought she was his wife. However, he was able to continue in his lifestyle until one weekend she received a call from the police to say her father had been found wandering in the village and could not remember where he lived. At this point she contacted the GP who was unable to provide a clear diagnosis. There were no clear referral pathways and they were referred to a number of different specialists before her father received a diagnosis of vascular dementia. At this point, the daughter had just settled her father into a care home when he suddenly deteriorated, attacked another resident and needed to be moved to a secure unit. She felt having a clearer diagnosis earlier on would have helped to prepare her for the changes in her father's behaviour and find more suitable accommodation at the outset.

Source: based on unpublished data, Brown Wilson (2007).

Many of the recommendations in Brooker et al. (2014) for a timely diagnosis refer to the importance of raising public awareness and reducing the stigma associated with dementia. A public health campaign in the United Kingdom (UK), initiated by the National Dementia Strategy entitled 'Living well with Dementia' (Department of Health, 2009) began this process. England, Northern Ireland, Scotland and Wales, subsequently developed localised strategies taking into account the local context of each nation. A key priority was to support people with dementia to remain in the community for longer providing appropriate support and services for the person with dementia and their caregiver. Many care organisations around the world provide web-based resources to people with dementia and their supporters providing a range of information with the aim of enabling decisions to be made by and with the person with dementia. Although there is still some way to go to raise public awareness, the recognition that dementia requires a global public health strategy is an important first step (WHO, 2015).

While most people say they would want to know if they had a diagnosis of dementia, many still receive the news with shock or disbelief (Bryden, 2002; Prince et al., 2011). However, not all people react negatively; for some a diagnosis brings a sense of relief and/or empowerment (Brooker et al., 2014). Reading the accounts of those who have been given a diagnosis suggest there are complex emotions involved (Bryden, 2015) which in turn require a range of supportive strategies to support people with dementia and those close to them in navigating the emotional responses that occur following diagnosis (Bryden, 2002). Christine Bryden (2002) speaks of the adaptive behaviours such as anxiety and depression that may be confused with the symptoms of dementia. It is important to see the person with dementia in a social context and understand their coping mechanisms before they had dementia to enable the professionals supporting them to make the distinction between dementia and adaptive behaviours. The focus at the point of diagnosis should be to enable the person with dementia to re-establish their wellbeing using psychotherapeutic approaches, not only pharmacological treatments (Bryden, 2002). This is particularly important when we consider the implications of younger people being diagnosed with dementia.

Myth 3: 'I am too young to have dementia'

There are no reliable prevalence figures of Young Onset Dementia worldwide (Rossor et al., 2010). It is thought that over 40,000 people in the UK live with Young Onset Dementia (Alzheimer's Society, 2014) and approximately 25,100 people in Australia (Australian Institute of Health and Welfare, 2012). Young Onset Dementia refers to people under the age of 65 as this age tends to signal the end of employment and the beginning of retirement. People as young as 30 may be diagnosed with a form of dementia and it is thought that the younger the person, the more likely there may be a genetic cause (Rossor et al., 2010). The figures for Young Onset Dementia represent a small percentage of people when compared with figures for those over 65 (Prince et al., 2015). However as dementia is considered something that happens primarily to older people, there is a substantial delay in time to diagnosis in this young onset group. In two prospective cohort studies in the Netherlands, the time to diagnosis of people with Young Onset Dementia exceeded that of late onset dementia by an average of 1.6 years (van Vliet et al., 2013). This may be due to the difficulty for community practitioners in recognising slowly evolving symptoms (Iliffe et al., 2006) and the fact that dementia may present differently in younger people (Rossor et al., 2010).

The needs of people living with Young Onset Dementia and their caregivers are very different to older people as at the ages of 30, 40 and 50 the person with dementia will be at different life stages. Many for example may have young families and/or employment and financial responsibilities that will increase strain within the family as the person with dementia becomes less able to fulfil their previous roles and responsibilities within the family. This creates additional strain, relational problems and conflict in families (Allen et al., 2009; van Vliet et al., 2010).

The impact of the diagnosis on the person with Young Onset Dementia was described in a UK-based phenomenological study involving eight participants (Clemerson et al., 2014). The participants in this study described their experience as situated in their life cycle and social context: feeling too young for the diagnosis and losing their adult competence resulted in a disruption to their life cycle. These people described three stages of coming to terms with their diagnosis: readjusting their self-identity; overcoming isolation through reconnection with those around them; and regaining a sense of control over their lives (Clemerson et al., 2014).

As the person with Young Onset Dementia may be a parent, this means the caregiving responsibilities within the family may fall to children as the other parent maintains or takes over the financial responsibilities within the family. In a prospective longitudinal study of 215 patient–caregiver dyads with Young Onset Dementia in the Netherlands, Bakker et al. (2013) found that informal care outstripped formal care by more than three times. Supervision/surveillance represented about 50% of the hours of informal care (approximately 230 hours/month) with much of this support provided by children under the age of 25. In this cohort, children described strain in relationships as the parent becomes less available for children with the child's role moving to that of a parent (Millenaar et al., 2014). Difficulties also emerged in coping with the different behaviours of their parent and many sought to avoid confrontation. Others coped by confiding in someone other than their healthy parent to avoid overburdening their parent. The help provided needed to be paced according to the children's needs, although most children appreciated the opportunity to speak with someone who knew their situation (Millenaar et al., 2014). Some of the issues experienced by families included the stigma associated with having a young parent with a diagnosis of dementia and lack of age appropriate services (Bakker et al., 2013).

The well known author and dementia advocate Christine Bryden, following diagnosis of early onset dementia, recounts how her diagnosis changed her relationships with her children as they took on the role of caregivers, with her eldest daughter deferring her university degree to remain close to the family (Bryden, 2015). Over time, Christine was able to redirect her abilities and passion to living well with dementia, becoming an advocate for others living with the condition. Most of Christine's experiences however are based on early experiences of frustration in trying to navigate the system with many different reactions and responses from healthcare professionals.

Myth 4: 'People with dementia cannot communicate'

One of the symptoms of many types of dementia is the loss of language as the dementia progresses. Christine Bryden (2015) writes eloquently about how she lost the thread of conversations and could not always remember the words she needed. There were times when she went along with people, because she could not find the words to explain why she didn't want to do something. This situation has the potential for people with dementia to withdraw from social situations where they feel unable to keep up and thus become isolated. This could happen in residential environments as well as in the community. As healthcare professionals, communicating with people living with dementia in hospitals or other residential environments is critical to ensure we are able to provide effective and safe care as a minimum requirement. Working with the belief that people with dementia are unable to communicate in meaningful ways is probably the most important barrier preventing good quality dementia care.

Practice scenario 1.2

I was conducting a series of workshops with colleagues in one care home in the UK (see Brown Wilson et al., 2013). The questionnaire that was given out at the beginning of the workshop demonstrated that very few staff believed people with dementia could communicate. During one of the workshops, a member of staff shared how she was beginning to have conversations with residents whom she thought were unable to communicate with her. Rather than focusing on the task of making the bed, while the resident with dementia was in the bathroom, the member of staff made the bed from the opposite side. This meant the resident in the bathroom could see the member of staff. The staff member then used the prompts from a memory box within the room to initiate a conversation. Using recognisable prompts enabled the person with dementia to lead the conversation about her life while the staff member simultaneously completed the task of making the bed.

Using prompts to communicate enables the person with dementia to be actively involved in the conversation as the above practice scenario suggests. When the topic of conversation is something that the person with dementia recognises then they are able to take the lead in a conversation. To facilitate a conversation such as this, it is important to avoid questions that relate to short-term memory that the person is unable to answer. For example, rather than asking if the person slept well or what they had for breakfast, you might comment that the person looks refreshed and ask them how they feel this morning.

There are clear ways of engaging people with dementia in ways that support them in being active partners in a conversation. The most important strategy is the pacing of information in a conversation, allowing time for people with dementia to consider the information and formulate a response. Don't assume they have not heard or do not understand simply because they are taking time to respond. Remove background noise and try to have important conversations in a quiet environment with minimal distractions. If you are speaking with a person with dementia make sure you can be seen; for example avoid sitting with your back to an open window as the light shining behind you will not allow the person with dementia to see the non-verbal cues they may use to follow the conversation. If the person with dementia loses the thread of the conversation, don't assume they are unable to understand. Gently rephrase what has been said so far to help them regain the thread. However avoid finishing sentences or finding words unless you are asked. If the person with dementia does not answer your question or if what they say appears out of context, acknowledge what they have said to encourage them to say more about their answer. Being patient and remaining calm with a positive tone to your voice are important ways of ensuring the person with dementia feels comfortable. Active listening is also an important part of communicating with a person living with dementia. This means maintaining eye contact, avoiding unnecessary or distracting gestures and repeating what you have heard back to the person to make sure you have understood their meaning.

People with dementia might not always retain the ability to communicate with spoken language, but this does not mean they lose the ability to communicate. As a person with dementia's ability to communicate verbally deteriorates, there are other forms of communication that family and professional caregivers may recognise such as a change in temperament or emotion when a certain course of action is followed. Behaviour is a powerful form of communication but it may not always be intentional and this is an important feature of the different forms of dementia. For this reason, it is vital that we, as healthcare professionals, don't make assumptions about types of behaviours. For example, damage to a person's brain means that they will not have the same level of control over responses as they once had, depending on the area of brain affected. In some types of dementia, this may be known, such as Frontotemporal dementia, which affects the part of the brain responsible for things such as personality, mood, social behaviour and self-control (Alzheimer's Australia, 2015). Understanding the context of the behaviour and the impact of the social and physical environment is also important.

As the dementia advances, it may appear that the person is no longer communicating, but it is at this point where other ways of making a connection are needed. This is not to say that we should stop speaking to the person with dementia; indeed, it is important to maintain that connection, speaking to people about their families, previous interests, engaging them with photos of things they may recall. Maintaining connection with a person with advanced dementia might also take the form of touch, smell, music or art. In my experience as a practitioner, the experience of touch through hand massage often showed visible changes in a person's facial experience and muscle tone, demonstrating recognition to this connection.

Activity 1.3 Reflection

Refer to the person with dementia from Activity 1.1.

- Describe a situation where there was effective communication with the person with dementia.
- What made this communication effective?
- Identify some of the key barriers to effective communication with people with dementia in this environment.
- How might they be removed to facilitate effective communication?

As dementia progresses, people with dementia may not be as able to be involved in conversation as they once were, struggling to follow what others are saying, particularly if there are hearing difficulties or multiple people conversing. This may contribute to the stereotype that people with dementia lose their ability to make decisions. In her most recent book, Christine Bryden discusses how her preferences and choices have changed over the years as she has altered her life to accommodate her changing abilities as the dementia progresses (Bryden, 2015). This demonstrates the importance of keeping people living with dementia connected with decision-making that affects their lives.

Myth 5: 'People with dementia cannot make decisions'

We have seen earlier in this chapter that progressive loss of problem solving and making judgements are symptoms of dementia (Table 1.1). These are important skills in the decision-making process. Even though people may have difficulty remembering or being part of a conversation, it does not mean they lose the capacity to think for themselves, to have their own opinions or continue to make decisions. It is important that everyone within society recognises that people with dementia are still able to be involved in decision-making. As cognition and the ability to problem solve may fluctuate, this means that professionals and those providing services may need to adopt a more flexible way of working to accommodate this fluidity of cognitive ability. If the person with dementia is assessed as not able to be involved in the decision, this may simply reflect the time of day the decision is being made, rather than the ability of the person with dementia. For example, it is important that issues such as tiredness and times of medication are taken into account. If a person's cognitive ability varies, this can prove frustrating for the person with dementia particularly when they have other periods of being able to think clearly and make decisions.

In the UK, the Mental Capacity Act 2005 provides clear guidance on how to assess capacity when a person has a diagnosis of dementia. Whilst it is becoming increasingly recognised by professional caregivers that people living with dementia are able to make a range of decisions that affect the person's immediate wellbeing, it is not as often recognised that the person living with dementia is also able to make more complex decisions. Before considering capacity, any difficulties in communication should be removed in the first instance. For example, in communication it is important to ensure the pace of the conversation enables the person with dementia to remain involved rather than moving too fast. If it is clear that the person living with dementia is not following the conversation, then either the information should be revisited, or the conversation moved to another time when they are more able to participate. Such challenges regarding communication may create anxiety for caregivers and families, so the needs of the family, especially those providing care, also need to be considered. This may mean speaking to the family alone to hear their concerns, which also provides an opportunity and time for the family to provide their opinions without exerting duress on the person with dementia. When a number of people are involved in a conversation and the person with dementia is not sure about something, they may simply agree as they may not want to appear that they don't understand. This situation may result in a decision being reached that excludes the person with dementia from the decision-making process, even though they are physically present. It is essential that professional healthcare workers identify situations where the person with dementia is not appropriately involved. This may occur when family members have different points of view to the person with dementia about the decisions being made. Families may also believe that the person with dementia is not able to be involved in decisions, with adult children being less likely to involve their parents with dementia in the decision-making process (Hirschman et al., 2005). Family caregivers' assessment of capacity may also influence how they involve the person with dementia in financial decisions (Tilse et al., 2005), if they restrict information and choices in everyday decisions (Samsi and Manthorpe, 2013) or whether they make decisions about care independently to the person with dementia (Hirschman et al., 2005). Decision-making is situation specific being influenced by the interaction between the person's condition and the situation (UK Mental Capacity Act 2005). Therefore the assessment of capacity is not a one-off event but something that needs to be revisited depending on the decisions being made.

People living with dementia may have difficulties making complex decisions about the future involving finances and may opt to involve a close relative or other person to manage their finances. When older people defer to family members or others to make decisions, this is known as decisional dependence (Tilse et al., 2005) and may manifest caregivers assuming responsibility for bill paying and investments (Moye and Marson, 2007). In a comprehensive study of assets management in Australia, family caregivers identified the increased time required in communicating complex information to the person with dementia, and the difficulties experienced when the person with dementia was not able to articulate their preferences (Setterlund et al., 2002). Although many families may be supporting their family member with financial decisions, not all families will have attained a Power of Attorney.

Power of Attorney means different things in different countries so it is prudent that all healthcare practitioners understand the legal definition in the country or state in which the older person is resident. There are generally two types of Power of Attorney:

- Power of Attorney – when you wish to give someone the power to make decisions while you still have the capacity.
- Lasting (or Enduring) Power of Attorney – when the person no longer has the capacity to make decisions or no longer wishes to make these decisions.

The Attorney is able to make decisions about finances, personal wellbeing and health and social care. This may include the disposal of assets, medical care, who can see the person, where they live and the care provided to the person, what they should eat, what kind of social activities the person can take part in. However, it is important to understand the presumption of capacity means that the person with dementia can still be involved in the decision-making process even when a Power of Attorney is in place.

Dementia often affects executive functions, such as remembering what items are for and/or planning out activities in a logical sequence to reach an end point. This may mean that activities involving remembering where you are going or how to get there become challenging. Decisions such as these also affect activities that enable people to remain independent – not being able to drive a car for example will have daily ramifications for a person's ability to engage with the world in their usual pattern of behaviour.

Being able to drive a car is a recognised lifestyle in many countries with the need to stop driving due to older age noted as a major life transition with poor outcomes on health and wellbeing (Liddle et al., 2014). Not being able to maintain an activity that was once taken for granted, such as driving, may undermine a person's sense of self. For this reason, people with dementia may not always elect to stop driving. On other occasions the person with dementia may lose insight into their abilities, which then makes it difficult to involve them in the decision-making process.

Jackie Liddle and colleagues (2014) identified the active role that family caregivers played in supporting the person with dementia to reach a decision about their need to stop driving, which ranged from implementing safety strategies such as accompanying the person with dementia or offering to drive, active negotiation, or conflict where the person with dementia blamed the family caregiver for not allowing them to continue driving (Liddle et al., 2014). While there may be similar patterns in the process of driving cessation between older drivers and those with dementia, there are also key differences (Liddle et al., 2014). A qualitative study exploring this issue used the perspectives of people living with dementia who were retired drivers, family caregivers and health professionals to identify three stages (see Figure 1.3).

Christine Bryden (2015) describes how she would use strategies such as only driving with someone in the car so they could direct her, until the day she came to drive and could not remember the process. At this point, she made the decision not to drive again. From the work conducted by Jackie Liddle and colleagues (2014), it is critical that conversations about issues such as driving are initiated at the early stages of dementia so that support for driving cessation can be individualised, sensitive and involve the person with dementia and their family (Liddle et al., 2014).

From this section we can see that assessment of capacity is considered situational and complex, dependent upon the interaction between the person's condition and the situation (Mental Capacity Act 2005). Therefore, this means that assessment of capacity needs to be revisited involving the person with dementia depending upon

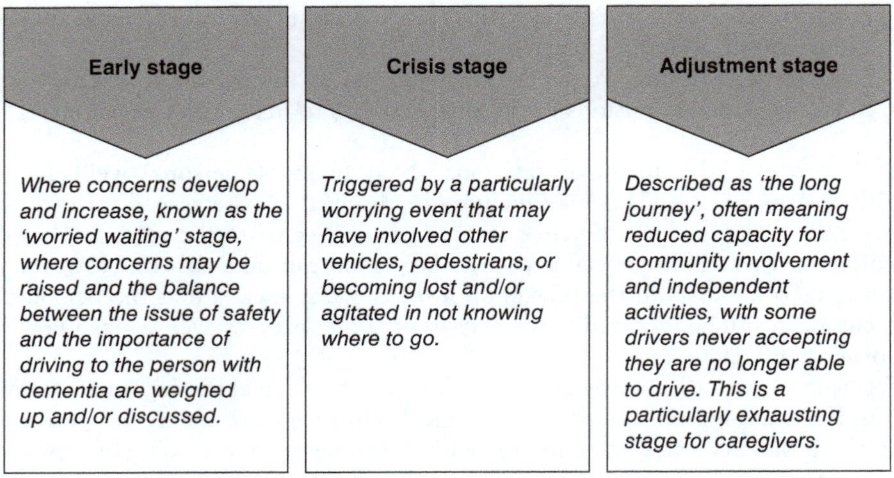

Early stage	Crisis stage	Adjustment stage
Where concerns develop and increase, known as the 'worried waiting' stage, where concerns may be raised and the balance between the issue of safety and the importance of driving to the person with dementia are weighed up and/or discussed.	*Triggered by a particularly worrying event that may have involved other vehicles, pedestrians, or becoming lost and/or agitated in not knowing where to go.*	*Described as 'the long journey', often meaning reduced capacity for community involvement and independent activities, with some drivers never accepting they are no longer able to drive. This is a particularly exhausting stage for caregivers.*

Figure 1.3 Stages of driving cessation, according to Liddle et al. (2013)

the decision being made. Advance care planning is an example of a decision that may need to be revisited as the person adapts to living with dementia.

Myth 6: 'Dementia is not a cause of death'

Dementia is a terminal condition and while we consider the value of living well with dementia, we must also consider the importance of a 'good death' with dementia. Palliative care should adopt a multidisciplinary approach, including the person with dementia, their family and friends. However, a recent report suggests that people with dementia have less access to quality palliative care services than those with other life limiting conditions such as cancer (Marie Curie Cancer Care with Alzheimer's Society, 2013). This may be due to the lack of understanding that dementia is a terminal condition and subsequently it may not always be identified on death certificates as the cause of death (Todd et al., 2013). In a consensus statement on behalf of the European Association for Palliative Care (EAPC), palliative care in dementia was seen as important with goals and priorities reflecting the progress of dementia from moderate through to advanced stages (van der Steen et al., 2014). In a review of educational initiatives for staff involved in providing palliative care for people with dementia, many identified the need for staff training but no studies found improvement in outcomes for people with dementia (Raymond et al., 2014a).

Advance Care Planning (ACP) is an important feature of supporting people with dementia to die with dignity, being offered care in a way they wish by those who know them. Advance care plans are generally written when a person has capacity to make these decisions and due to their legal status can support decision-makers in identifying when to seek medical attention in the later stages of dementia. ACP is a dynamic process of recording a person's preferences of care and if opted for should be started whilst the person with dementia retains capacity to enable person-centred care (Exley et al., 2009). This means that conversations about the end of life need to be approached in the early stages of dementia, whilst people with dementia are still able to be actively engaged in the decision-making process (Marie Curie Cancer Care with Alzheimer's Society, 2013). In a systematic review of the literature on ACP and dementia only three studies were located, all of which were in residential aged care facilities (Robinson et al., 2012). Many people with dementia in this context were not judged to have the capacity to enter into ACP, suggesting that waiting until admission to Residential Aged Care Facilities (RACF) might be too late. However, when ACP was introduced, into RACF, there was a reduction in hospitalisation and an increase in hospice use at the end of life (Robinson et al., 2012). Overall, it has been quite challenging to convince older people to make Advance Care Plans which often leaves the decisions towards the end of life to family members and staff (Samsi and Manthorpe, 2011).

It is often problematic to predict when a person with dementia is coming to the end of their life. However, a number of signs and symptoms may be indicators that the end of life is drawing closer. These include deterioration of speech and needing help with everyday activities; increasing difficulty in walking, standing and controlling the head; difficulties in eating and swallowing; bladder and bowel incontinence (Alzheimer's Society, 2013). At this point in time, it is critical to involve caregivers and families, enabling them to remain part of the decision-making process, especially when the person with dementia is no longer able to communicate. However, the views of caregivers of people dying with dementia are diverse (Raymond et al., 2014b). In a consensus statement on behalf of the European Association for Palliative Care (van der Steen et al., 2014), person-centred care, communication and shared decision-making were seen as the main priorities when providing palliative care for people with dementia. In the following chapter, we will explore how to implement person-centred care for people living with dementia.

Conclusion

This chapter has considered the myths associated with dementia from the perspective of the person living and dying with dementia, their family caregivers and those staff that support them. We have considered each of these myths in context to the value of timely diagnosis considering the critical nature of involving the person with dementia and their families at each point of the journey. Recognising the terminal nature of dementia means that we may need to adopt a different approach in supporting people with the condition and their families, ensuring they are able to make and record their decisions at each point of the journey. However, there may be times when decision-making is neither easy nor straightforward: for example, we have considered financial decisions and the issue of driving as examples where support by professionals may be required. A thread through this chapter has been the notion of person-centred care as a mechanism for ensuring the involvement of people with dementia and their families throughout the journey of dementia. What person-centred care means in dementia care will be critically explored in more detail in the following chapter.

Final reflection

Dementia is a progressive condition based on myriad diseases that ultimately leads to the death of the person. Each of these diseases progresses differently and so will affect people in different ways. This means that each person's experience of dementia will be unique and affected by a range of factors including the myths and stereotypes they have come into contact with. When professionals who meet the person with dementia and their supporters in the early stages of this condition subscribe to negative stereotypes or commonly held myths, this will impact greatly on these initial experiences. Dementia has been equated with a journey which we as professionals may embark on alongside the person with dementia and their families. This book is part of that journey as we consider how best to work with the person with dementia and their families.

Further reading

Social Care Institute for Excellence Dementia Gateway

This Dementia Gateway provides a range of resources starting with a brief video that supports us in understanding the nature of the condition. Available at: www.scie.org.uk/dementia/about/ (accessed 26/01/17).

Communication

DEEP (Dementia Engagement and Empowerment Project) *Guide: Dementia Words Matter*. This guide provides an overview of the importance of language from the perspective of the person living with dementia. This is particularly important in relation to people living with young onset dementia. Available at: www.youngDementiauk.org/sites/default/files/DEEP-Guide-Language.pdf (accessed 26/01/17).

Young Onset Dementia

Younger Onset Dementia: A Practical Guide was developed in Australia and has been adopted in the UK to support professionals with supporting those with young onset dementia. Available at: www.fightdementia.org.au/publications/quality-dementia-care

The following website provides personal stories of people's individual journeys with dementia: www.youngDementiauk.org/personal-stories-0 (accessed 26/01/17).

Supporting people with dementia to take risks

Nothing Ventured, Nothing Gained: Risk Guidance for People with Dementia (Department of Health, 2010).

This document moves from a focus on Risk Management to a Risk Enablement Strategy with clear guidance on how to achieve this. The document also provides a range of evidence on areas covered in this chapter such as driving and finance. Available at: www.gov.uk/government/uploads/system/uploads/attachment_data/file/215960/dh_121493.pdf (accessed 10/09/16).

Power of Attorney and what it means

Age UK is a useful source on this topic. Available at: www.ageuk.org.uk/money-matters/legal-issues/powers-of-attorney/lasting-power-of-attorney/ (accessed 26/01/17).

Maintaining a healthy brain

Your Brain Matters is part of an awareness raising campaign in Australia providing simple messages on how to ensure brain health. The following link provides access to a range of evidence-based resources including a link to the BrainyApp: www.yourbrainmatters.org.au/a-little-help/download-information (accessed 26/01/17).

2

Developing relationship-based approaches to dementia care

Learning objectives

By the end of this chapter, the reader will be able to:

- Critically consider the different relationship-based approaches to care and how they form a continuum of practice.
- Analyse the differences between individualised, person-centred and relationship-centred care.
- Examine how the use of biography can be used to implement relationship-based approaches to care.
- Investigate how you might implement person-centred and relationship-centred care in your practice.

Introduction

In the previous chapter we considered a range of myths that impact on the journey of the person with dementia and those important to them, from diagnosis through to death. The discussion demonstrated the value of healthcare professionals understanding how dementia affects a person and the potential for treatment and support as the condition progresses. Dementia has been likened to a journey that affects everyone differently and may take an individual to different places depending on their life experience, their personality and the type of dementia they are experiencing. Supporting people with dementia and those that care for them requires a focus on a range of relationships. In my first book *Caring for Older People: A Shared Approach*, I outlined three approaches to care based on my research that focused on relationships between older people, staff and families: individualised, person-centred and relationship-centred (Brown Wilson, 2012). I use the term relationship-based approaches to describe an approach that requires the development of positive relationships with the person, their family and other staff members. In my early research, I observed the same staff adopting three different approaches, individualised, person-centred and relationship-centred, for different people at different times. Those observations have been used to develop a continuum of care along which each approach is based. This means that there may be times when we, as professional caregivers, may focus on individualised care but then move to a more person-centred approach when the context enables this. This moves our practice away from the 'all or nothing' argument, where staff working in dementia care feel they do not have the time to implement person-centred care. In this chapter we will examine different approaches to care and how they might be implemented. We will discuss individualised, person-centred and relationship-centred care, reviewing the differences, the evidence and application of each approach. The key argument proposed in this chapter is that as we get to know a person, we understand the stories being shared with us about their life experiences, which can then be integrated into the everyday care routines for that person, whether they are in a hospital environment, or live in their own home, assisted living or long-term residential environments. Irrespective of the location, the value of relationships in care provision remains a consistent imperative in ensuring the quality of effective and meaningful care for people with dementia. Retaining this emotional connection becomes vital to the person with dementia as their ability to communicate alters.

What do we mean by a continuum of care?

As nurses and healthcare practitioners, we may adopt a model of care that the organisation in which we work dictates. At the same time, we ourselves have a worldview of what it means to provide care or to be a 'professional caregiver'. If the two approaches do not reflect each other, there can often be tension that affects our overall job satisfaction. Students who seek to implement theoretical models of care often report a tension between what they are learning and the pressures exerted by the environment that constrains how they practise. This means many students and early career practitioners become encultured into the way the organisation wishes to deliver care, without examining other ways of working. The concept of a continuum of care provides you with the flexibility of being able to meet the competing demands of a busy environment whilst practising with a focus on relationships when supporting people living with dementia. I have adopted the concept of a continuum to describe a range from individualised developing to person-centred and on to relationship-centred care. There are gradual changes that might occur in your practice that enable you to progress from an individualised approach to person-centred care and then on to relationship-centred care – and this may be context specific and therefore different for everyone. Equally, there might be times when you need to return to an individualised focus and this is also acceptable as it means that you can return to adopting person-centred care when the context enables you to do so. Before we can understand how the continuum works, we need to consider what each approach means and how we implement relationship-based approaches in everyday practice.

Individualised care

Individualised care was initially considered as an antidote to task-centred care, where the focus was primarily on meeting the needs of the organisation and meant that the needs of older people or those with dementia were seen as secondary to the needs of the organisation. There has been a cultural shift over the past two decades with a greater focus on addressing the needs of the person with dementia.

Activity 2.1 Critical thinking

Explain how you might implement individualised care in an organisation where you are currently practising:

- Write down how you provide choices for the people you are caring for.
- What are these choices related to?
- How do you know about these choices?
- Are these choices unique to this person; if so how?
- What are the areas that are common to many people?
- How does this influence the management of your care?
- Are there any choices you are unable to accommodate – why is this?

There have been some concerns raised that people implementing individualised care confuse this with person-centred care in dementia environments (Brooker and Latham, 2015). A helpful distinction might be to consider the focus of individualised care as remaining focused on the task. Returning to Activity 2.1, consider if all of the choices are related to a task of care that needs to be delivered for that person. Whilst adopting an individualised approach takes into consideration an individual's likes/dislikes and choices, they remain focused on how we as practitioners can deliver safe and effective care that meets the identified needs of the individual. This is not poor care but was described in my research study (Brown Wilson, 2007) as the minimum standard of care that older people and families wish to receive. For example, where I observed an individualised approach to care, staff were highly motivated to do a good job and often defined this in terms of the task of care and how they were able to achieve this whilst still promoting the choices of the individual (Figure 2.1). However, we also know that choice is often provided within the confines of what the organisation is prepared to deliver and the level of deviation from the accepted norm that the organisation is prepared to permit. Returning to Activity 2.1, consider when you have not been able to deliver on the choices of an individual – why is this? When you are not able to deliver on the choices of an individual this is generally due to competing needs of the organisation. However, when we do not deliver individualised care, we could say we are falling below the minimum standard that older people and families view as acceptable care. Certainly in my research, there were times when individualised care was necessary such as

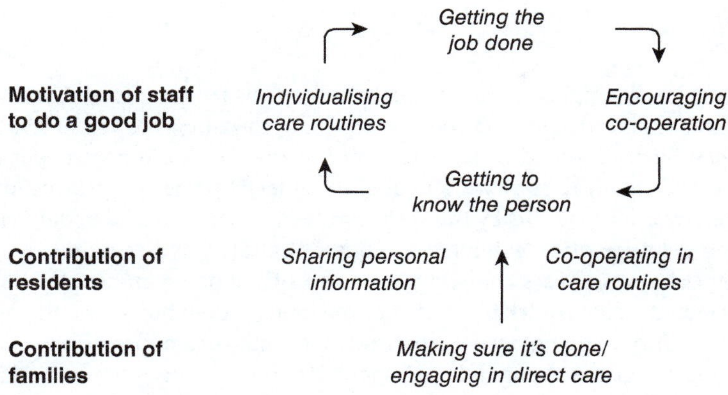

Figure 2.1 Individualised care

when new staff were starting and didn't know the people they were supporting or when a person was initially admitted to the environment in which staff are working. In this context, we can view individualised care as a starting point on a continuum of care where the focus is on ensuring good quality care and using care routines as an opportunity to get to know the person.

One of the concerns staff and students have shared with me over the years has been that they often feel unable to deliver person-centred care all of the time and so they tend to revert to a focus on the task with the belief that they don't have time to implement person-centred care. However, I have seen staff adopt different approaches to care at different times of the day depending on whom they are working with and who they are supporting. In this context, the staff move between individualised and person-centred care working within the constraints of the organisation. However, many staff may still find themselves working alongside staff with different values and motivations and so may need to adopt a level of flexibility in how care is delivered as part of an overall team. Staff who described their motivation as being able to deliver good care also listened to the stories shared by residents and their families that enabled them to provide individualised care. Therefore, individualised care could be conceptualised as a starting point on a continuum, to ensure the focus remains on good quality care alongside using care routines to get to know the person (Brown Wilson and Davies, 2009).

Practice scenario 2.1

Beatrice had been an English teacher and had won prizes for her grasp of language and spelling in particular. Her husband Rodger recounted the first holiday when he realised something was wrong when his wife started asking him how to spell words for the postcards she was writing. When he looked at the postcards, the words did not

(Continued)

(Continued)

make any sense. At this point, they began to make plans for the future. When I met her, Beatrice had advanced dementia and was unable to communicate verbally. There were times when Beatrice would whisper to staff but the words did not appear to make any sense and then the staff were unable to understand her, so Beatrice would go quiet. There was a consensus by the staff that Beatrice did not understand what was happening. Beatrice often exhibited a range of agitated and repetitive behaviours that meant she was always changing seats and sitting down on people already in a seat. She would walk in quick bursts out of the lounge room but would not appear to know where she was going once she had left. She would often turn off the light when she left the lounge room engendering shouts from other residents and staff still in that room. Staff told me Beatrice had been a teacher and they were able to recount what Beatrice liked to eat, how she liked to dress and how she preferred her hygiene needs to be met. Her husband Rodger would visit every 2–3 days in the afternoon. Just before Rodger's visit, Beatrice would become very agitated but on his arrival Beatrice would sit or walk with him and could often be seen to move to sit on his lap. After the visit, Beatrice would routinely sit quietly for up to an hour in the lounge room. On one afternoon, I noticed Beatrice had been physically restrained to a chair by a small table. I asked why this was the case as it was about the same time Rodger would usually visit. Staff informed me that Rodger was not visiting this afternoon and Beatrice had become so agitated that the staff had feared for her safety. They had undertaken a risk assessment for physical restraint and considered this was the best option. Rodger had told me that he and Beatrice would often walk in a local country park and watch the ducks, which was an activity they had shared for many years. Beatrice had loved the outdoors and had been an avid gardener.

Source: from Brown Wilson (2007), unpublished data.

Staff caring for Beatrice were highly motivated to 'do a good job' and they often defined good quality care as meeting the needs of people in ways that reflected their likes, dislikes and choices they might have made prior to moving into the care home. Staff could identify Beatrice's likes and dislikes about the food and her dress and how they responded to these preferences. For example, one staff member explained that Beatrice's annoying habit of turning the light off every time she left the lounge room could be explained by the fact she had been a teacher and would have always been the last person out of the room and so would always have turned off the light. Understanding the significance of Beatrice's action I believe was the first step in moving towards person-centred care as this staff member understood the significance of the action for Beatrice. The key difference here was the recognition that this was more than a random behaviour but had significance in relation to Beatrice's life history. Since Beatrice was unable to verbally share this information, staff relied on the family contribution of sharing stories about Beatrice's life. Without the contribution of families, staff would not be able to individualise dementia care in the same way.

Recognition of a significant behaviour is a necessary first step in person-centred care but by itself is not sufficient to change the focus of care. This information now needs to be applied in ways that promote the identity of the person, developing insight into details that are significant to the person with dementia.

Person-Centred Care

Person-centred care is becoming increasingly synonymous with good quality care. Person-centred dementia care is based on the philosophy of Professor Tom Kitwood, whose pioneering work articulates how personhood is conferred to a person with dementia by the social responses and environment in which the person is located:

> a standing or status that is bestowed on one human being, by others, in the context of relationship and social being. It implies recognition, respect and trust. (Kitwood, 1997: 8)

'Dementia reconsidered' (Kitwood, 1997) challenged the medical model and prevailing culture of dementia care by considering the viewpoint of the person with dementia. Professor Tom Kitwood identified that people with dementia have five overlapping needs which will be influenced by the environment in which they are cared for and the relationship with those who care for them (see Figure 2.2). Kitwood suggested a way forward for dementia care that proposed to make staff aware of how their actions worked against the wellbeing of people with dementia often unintentionally. He based this work on the idea of a 'malignant social psychology' that often robbed

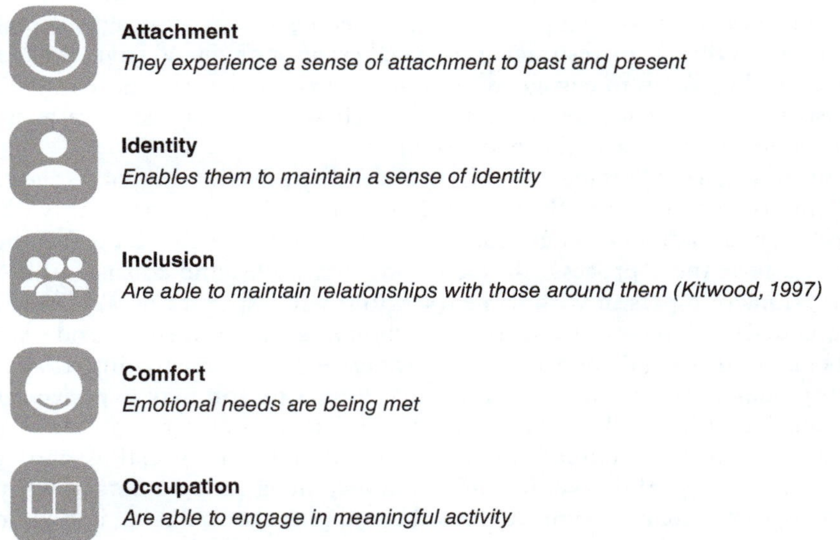

Figure 2.2 Five needs of a person living with dementia, based on Kitwood (2007)

people with dementia of their self-esteem, confidence and eventually their personhood (Kitwood, 1997).

The person with dementia is more likely to experience a greater sense of wellbeing when each of these domains are considered in their care (Figure 2.2).

Activity 2.2 Critical Thinking

Using Practice scenario 2.1, identify how Beatrice's needs might have been met using Kitwood's principles in Figure 2.2.

Beatrice's need for:	What was done	What could have been done differently
Attachment		
Identity		
Inclusion		
Comfort		
Occupation		

Using Kitwood's principles above, you would have interpreted Beatrice's behaviour as communicating an emotional need. For example, when Beatrice was trying to sit on other residents' laps, you might have considered this as missing her husband, so you might have suggested you could sit and hold Beatrice's hand, so she felt an emotional attachment at that point in time. When Beatrice was engaged in repetitive behaviours, rather than restraining, a member of staff might have walked with Beatrice in the garden to engage in meaningful activity that she has enjoyed in the past, so maintaining her sense of identity. These ideas suggest a very different approach to Beatrice's actual experience of care.

Dementia Care Mapping (DCM) was developed as a way of assessing the wellbeing of the person with dementia and the interaction they had with their environment and others using a coded observational schedule. DCM can be used both as a tool and a process (Brooker and Surr, 2006) and consists of in-depth observations of a person with dementia with their responses of wellbeing or ill-being coded at intervals (BSI, 2010). Observers are trained to code signs of wellbeing or ill-being demonstrated by the person with dementia into time frames that provide an overall impression of how long a person may experience either wellbeing or ill-being. In addition to this, actions from care workers are also recorded. Actions that fall into the categories of malignant social psychology are described as personal detractors and could include ignoring a person when they are trying to attract attention. Actions that support the wellbeing of people with dementia are described as personal enhancers and could include validating the experience of the person with dementia. As a process, feedback to staff occurs following the observation with suggested actions agreed and a follow-up observation undertaken (Chenoweth et al., 2009). Examples of these actions are included in the feedback as ways that caregivers are dealing well with certain situations or issues that may need to be improved, which in turn enhance the experience of both the person with dementia and those caring for them (Rokstad et al., 2013). Kitwood's approach has been considered important for relocating the person with dementia as central to dementia care.

The legacy of Tom Kitwood remains central to the provision of person-centred dementia care as more organisations are now considering how to implement person-centred care as a mechanism to improve the quality of care. A reflection of this progress is that policy documents now refer to person-centred care (National Collaborating Centre for Mental Health, 2007). One criticism in the literature has been a lack of detail in how people might implement person-centred care (Dewing, 2004). Dawn Brooker (2004) has subsequently developed Kitwood's theory of person-centred care into four key principles for practice, the VIPS Framework, being: V = Values and promotes the rights of the person; I = provides individualised care according to needs; P = understands care from the Perspective of the person with dementia; S = supportive Social psychology and social environment that enables the person to remain in relationship to others. An expert consensus group has identified a range of indicators grouped around the domains of VIPS enabling organisations to assess how they achieve each domain (Brooker and Latham, 2015). For example, a day care service used this model to evaluate its service demonstrating an achievement of above good quality in every indicator and excellence in 83% of the indicators (Association for Dementia Studies (ADS), 2010) with the conclusion that:

> The service is an exemplar of positive person-centred dementia care. The staff team are passionately committed to ensuring that all the people with dementia who attend the centre have a high quality service, which meets their individual needs, promotes their abilities and enhances their wellbeing. (ADS, 2010: 9)

The VIPS Framework has been used in a range of projects to support services in achieving person-centred care alongside the development of training materials (Brooker and Latham, 2015). An early example was in the Enriched Opportunities Programme (EOP) which used these principles in extra care housing and care homes. This approach was a multi-level intervention that focused on an activities-based approach to care (Brooker and Woolley, 2007). Each of the development sites identified a senior person, known as an EOP Locksmith, who was responsible for identifying residents' needs and developing a strategy for person-centred care as well as being responsible for changing practice to ensure the implementation of person-centred care (Brooker and Woolley, 2007). Direct care staff were also engaged to be more involved in the fun activities, which encouraged them to see the ability of the person with dementia (Brooker and Woolley, 2007). Overall, this programme demonstrated statistically significant improvements in wellbeing and depression scores alongside an increase in diversity of activity for many residents. It is important to note that these study sites were already nursing homes providing good quality care and were interested in being part of the research (Brooker et al., 2007). However, this study demonstrates that it is possible to provide person-centred care in an organisation and subsequently improve outcomes for people living with dementia.

Person-centred care may mean different things in different environments, so it is important to consider how person-centred care is implemented and how this might transfer to improved outcomes for the person with dementia. The VIPS Practice Model (VPM) was developed to support the implementation of person-centred care in residential aged care facilities in Norway to support staff to focus on the interactions between staff, the person with dementia and the environment (Rosvik et al., 2013). VPM includes a clear structure:

- A weekly consensus meeting (45 minutes–1 hour) with a set structure and set roles and functions in the team.
- Staff training underpinned with a manual with practical knowledge and examples of PCC, non-pharmacological treatment related to each indicator in the VIPS framework and assessment tools.
- Supportive management that formed a PCC expertise group common for the whole institution consisting of four experienced senior staff to be available to support the staff on request (Rosvik et al., 2011).
- A Registered Nurse responsible for speaking with the person with dementia and the family to find out about their life history and how this might impact on behaviours and emotions, becoming the coach for other staff and using this knowledge to support a change in care (Rosvik et al., 2013).

Rokstad and colleagues (2013) compared VPM to Dementia Care Mapping and education alone involving 624 people with dementia living in residential environments in Norway. Only 446 people completed the final assessments and there were no statistically significant results for behaviours or quality of life although there were promising results for depression (Rokstad et al., 2013).

Lyn Chenoweth and colleagues in Australia have also developed a person-centred model based on Tom Kitwood's principles (Chenoweth et al., 2009, 2014). Caring for Aged Dementia Care Resident Study (CADRES) compared person-centred care (PCC) to DCM and usual care. Staff were observed to be implementing PCC (Chenoweth et al., 2009) in the following ways:

- Attending to the person's feelings, experiences and perceptions of that person's own reality.
- Attending to the person's emotional, social, physical and spiritual needs and establishing positive relationships.
- Assisting and encouraging the person to maintain function and engage in meaningful life experiences.
- Creating an enriched environment.
- Avoiding triggers for distress.

An interesting observation from this study was that few care plans in the study described the care delivered (Chenoweth et al., 2009). This raises an interesting point in how staff may implement PCC but find it difficult to document how this is achieved. These interventions significantly reduced agitation in both the PCC and DCM groups (Chenoweth et al., 2009) although there were no statistically significant outcomes for staff burnout or health (Jeon et al., 2012). The costs were calculated taking into account staff time in dealing with agitation and demonstrated a cost saving per resident for the behaviours averted through person-centred care (Chenoweth et al., 2009). Further work by this team in the PerCen study (Chenoweth et al., 2014) demonstrated a statistically significant difference in both agitation and quality of life for people living with dementia with 59% of staff implementing PCC.

The studies reviewed so far demonstrate the difficulty in identifying measurable outcomes that can be influenced by positive relationships and wellbeing experienced by the person with dementia. Lyn Chenoweth and colleagues used large randomised controlled trials to demonstrate a reduction in need-driven dementia-compromised agitation and the associated costs in staff time when individually tailored solutions were developed (Chenoweth et al., 2009, 2014). This provides us with a promising direction in how we might not only implement relationship based approaches to care but also identify the benefits these approaches bring to the person with dementia and staff.

The research I conducted in residential environments in the UK adopted an inductive qualitative approach where I observed how different staff enacted the care routines and interacted with older people, including those with dementia, families and other staff (Brown Wilson, 2007). Using observation and interviews with residents, families and staff across three residential aged care facilities I was able to identify how staff enacted person-centred care (see Figure 2.3). Staff shared why they adopted different practices and what motivated their care which contributed to the detailed nature of the care interactions that enabled positive relationships leading to person-centred care and relationship-centred care (Brown Wilson and Davies, 2009; Brown Wilson et al., 2009).

If we return to the idea of a continuum of care, moving from individualised to person-centred care we are moving from knowing what routines to implement to understanding why these routines hold significance for that person and consequently making a decision to implement the details that matter to the person with dementia. Staff who enacted person-centred care in this way described a motivation to deliver

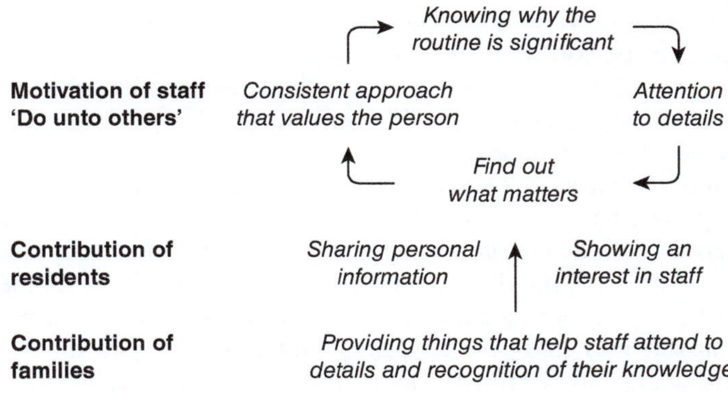

Figure 2.3 Person-centred care

the care they knew the person wanted because they would like someone to do that for them when they were in that position (Brown Wilson, 2009). When I observed person-centred care in action, the contribution of families was evident in helping out with little things that took up staff time, such as tidying up clothes so they were easier to find, or helping with the afternoon tea trolley. Older people themselves would also share stories that were imbued with symbolism or recount important life events. When a person with dementia was unable to continue sharing stories, families would take on this role.

Practice scenario 2.2

One evening I was spending time with staff and a family member when her father, who was a retired cattle farmer with dementia suddenly announced he had to 'get the cows in and shut the gate'. The daughter explained how she had told the staff about her father's past routine so they understood this behaviour. The staff member said she knew this background information and subsequently the routine in the care home was to explain the cows were already in and offer the gentleman a cup of tea as this was what would have happened after he had 'closed the gate'. This approach recognised that being a farmer was still an important aspect of this person's identity and rather than remind him he was in a care home, the staff would seek to maintain that identity by continuing the same routine he was used to in his own home.

We can see from Practice scenario 2.2 that families play an important role in contributing important information and supporting staff to understand the significance of behaviours when connected to previous routines. Not all people living with dementia have families. Staff in one dementia facility I was supporting described how they had looked at photos displayed in one resident's room to see how she had dressed before she had dementia. In every photo there had been jewellery and the staff made the effort to ensure each day that this resident was wearing her jewellery as this had been an important part of this woman's identity. These staff also recounted how not everyone attended to this important detail and that it can be dependent upon the person who is delivering care. Person-centred care demonstrates a consistent approach that values the person, which needs to be applied across shifts and teams and we will be exploring what this means in later chapters.

We saw earlier that meaningful activity is also an important element of person-centred care and this aspect can sometimes be lost in the care routines. Knowing that people liked gardening or enjoyed doing housework are all important ways of supporting people with dementia in maintaining meaningful activity. In one home I visited, a staff cleaner told me that one of the women would always come up and ask if she could help her in her cleaning and she would be given a cloth to help. We discovered that this lady had been a professional cleaner before she had developed dementia. Knowing this enabled the staff cleaner to engage the resident in conversation during the time the resident was helping her.

Person-centred care focuses on the person and what is important to the person, taking into account the contribution of the families and staff (Figure 2.3). Within residential environments there are often competing demands where staff tell me that it is difficult to routinely implement person-centred care. In considering the approaches I have outlined, person-centred care can be an extension of the care routines and when embedded within them, can promote a sense of wellbeing for the person with dementia. In my research (Brown Wilson and Davies, 2009), I observed teams of staff that worked in a way that enabled them to balance these competing demands and address the needs of staff and families. This was described as relationship-centred care.

Relationship-Centred Care

Relationship-centred care is the third approach I observed that moved from a focus on the person to a focus on relationships, considering the needs of all stakeholders in the relationship. This approach understood that there would be times when both family caregivers and staff would also have needs that might need to be considered within the relationship. Relationship-centred care (see Figure 2.4) is the final approach along the continuum of care we discussed at the beginning of this chapter.

Relationships in healthcare practice have been described as central to the therapeutic encounter (Tresolini et al., 1994). This concept challenges a purely biological approach to healthcare through consideration of the significance of the relationships between practitioners and those they care for as well as the communities within which they practise (Tresolini et al., 1994). Relationship-centred care is based on a therapeutic relationship which should have as its foundation a shared understanding

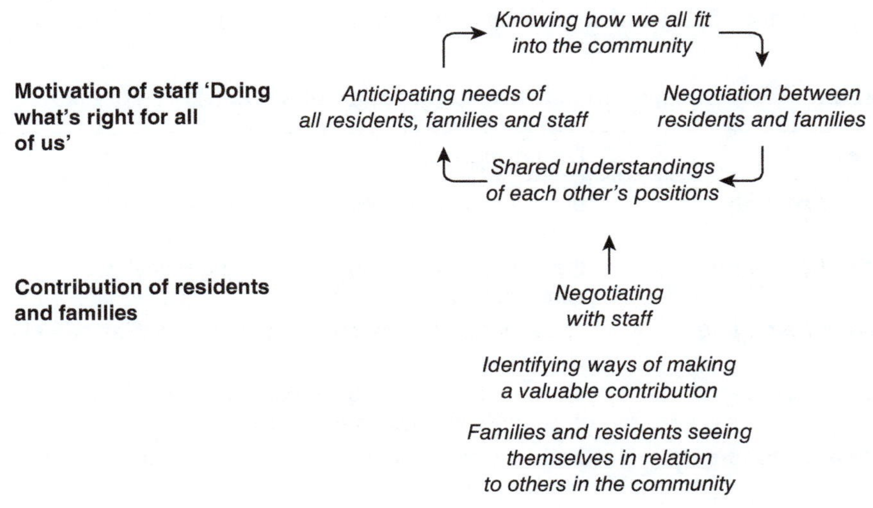

Figure 2.4 Relationship-centred care

of what health and illness means to the person and those close to them, in the context of the community in which they live. Relationship-centred care goes beyond the holistic person-centred model to consider relationships between other practitioners as well as between the person and their community:

> Practitioners' relationships with their patients, their communities and other practitioners are central to health care and are a vehicle for putting into action a new paradigm of health that integrates caring, healing and community. These relationships form the context within which people are helped to maintain their functioning and grow in the face of changes within themselves and their environment. (Tresolini et al., 1994: 24)

Using the principles of relationship-centred care, Professor Mike Nolan and his team (Nolan et al., 2001) developed the Senses Framework in response to a lack of a clear therapeutic direction for the care of older people (Table 2.1).

The term 'Senses' was chosen to reflect the subjective and perceptual nature of what determines 'good care' for both older people and staff, supporting the development of therapeutic relationships. The subjective nature of the 'Senses' would suggest that different contexts and interventions could create the 'Senses' for people in different ways (Nolan et al., 2004). It is proposed that when staff, older people, and their families experience the 'Senses' an enriched environment for care is created where positive relationships may develop (Nolan et al., 2006a). Ryan et al. (2008) described how staff demonstrated that the 'Senses' also provide a mechanism for how good relationships develop within dementia care triads in an organisation delivering community-based respite care. On the one hand, staff would look at the biography of a person with dementia and then identify an activity they might enjoy. The caregivers however were always informed about the activity and asked their opinion. This promoted a sense of continuity for both the person with dementia and their carer whilst promoting a sense of achievement for the staff that they were doing something meaningful and so making a difference. In this way, Mike Nolan and his

Table 2.1 The Senses Framework – after Nolan et al. (2001)

Senses	Description
Sense of security	of feeling safe and receiving or delivering competent and sensitive care
Sense of continuity	the recognition of biography, using the past to contextualise the present
Sense of belonging	opportunities to form meaningful relationships or feel part of a team
Sense of purpose	opportunities to engage in purposeful activities or to have a clear set of goals to aspire to
Sense of achievement	achieving meaningful or valued goals or to feel satisfied with one's efforts
Sense of significance	to feel that you matter, and that you are valued as a person

team argue that relationship-centred care attends to the needs of everyone in the relationship (Ryan et al., 2008). Nolan et al. (2004) argue that respect for personhood underpins positive relationships and Clare Surr (2006) concluded that relationships with staff, other residents and families were able to both promote or undermine the sense of self for a person with dementia (Surr, 2006).

The complexity of a relationship and understanding the needs of everyone in the relationship is challenging. In the observations and interviews referred to in the previous section (Brown Wilson, 2007) I observed how staff used the biographical knowledge from person-centred care to anticipate the needs of the person and then engage in negotiation to ensure the needs of everyone in the relationship (residents, families and staff) were met. This resulted in shared understandings and a sense of community (Figure 2.4). Practice scenario 2.3 provides an example where all of these relationships were taken into account to improve the experience of all residents, staff and the family member.

Practice scenario 2.3

Mr Au was an older man who would often move around the ward area, going up to people and trying to touch them. Other people and staff became very agitated with him and would try to make him stop, which resulted in aggressive behaviour both from Mr Au and other people towards Mr Au. The family of Mr Au never visited and staff drew the conclusion that he wasn't cared about. In workshops I was conducting with staff, I suggested that contacting the family might help explain this behaviour. The staff contacted his daughter to discuss Mr Au's behaviour. She told the staff her father used to volunteer in a Buddhist temple and would walk around the temple blessing people and she thought her father was following this routine. The staff then told the other residents in the ward that Mr Au was blessing them and all the other residents accepted this gesture. The staff began to accept this behaviour and Mr Au no longer displayed aggression. Initiating this dialogue with Mr Au's daughter enabled the daughter to build a relationship of trust with the staff as they began to contact her more regularly. Mr Au's daughter then disclosed that her father had attacked her with a knife before he was admitted to the ward and she was very frightened of him, which is why she did not visit. The staff then worked with Mr Au's daughter to enable her to understand the dementia and provided a supportive environment where she felt safe to visit her father.

If we consider relationship-centred care using Figure 2.4, we can see that once the staff recognised the significance of the routine for Mr. Au, they were able to anticipate that this activity would upset other people on the ward. Staff then explained the context of Mr. Au's behaviour to other residents, contributing to shared understandings. Staff now recognised how Mr. Au was contributing to the community within the ward. Staff also recognised that they also needed to focus on the needs of the daughter to enable her to contribute to her father's care.

Activity 2.3 Critical thinking

Using Table 2.1 identify how each of the senses were being created for Mr Au, his daughter and staff.

Sense	Person with dementia	Family member or significant other	Staff
Sense of security			
Sense of continuity			
Sense of belonging			
Sense of purpose			
Sense of achievement			
Sense of significance			

Relationships within health and social care environments are generally developed through care and daily living routines for which people may need support (Brown Wilson and Davies, 2009). As we have seen throughout this chapter, routines can be the vehicle by which staff are able to develop knowledge about a person's biography; this is the first step in being able to identify meaningful activity that is relevant to different people. Being able to engage in meaningful activity is a key part of feeling a sense of belonging and a sense of purpose (Nolan et al., 2006a). A person with dementia who sees their role in the care home as 'working' or 'helping staff' is able to maintain their sense of self when the role is recognised and valued by others (Surr, 2006). I propose that recognising meaningful activity promotes a sense of community where everyone's contributions are valued (Brown Wilson, 2009). Meaningful activity in helping out in the life of the home is becoming more common for those who wish to maintain roles they may have had in their own home and contributes to an overall sense of community (Owen, 2006). People with dementia can make a contribution to the community in different ways and understanding the biography of a person with dementia supports staff in enabling that person to maintain an important role, as Practice scenario 2.4 indicates.

Practice scenario 2.4

Staff would bring the laundry up to the lounge room each afternoon to fold and Heather would tell the other women that she had to help the staff now and move across to take her place at the table. She would talk to the staff while she was helping fold the laundry. She was often animated and spoke to the staff about her experiences as a younger woman. One day I noticed Heather wasn't participating and asked the staff why this might be and was told that Heather was feeling tired. Heather had told the staff she needed a 'day off'. Staff told me that this was an activity that Heather initiated on most days because she took pride in being able to do housework as this had been her role all of her married life. Heather told me that she was helping staff and this was her job. She spoke with a sense of pride when speaking about this.

Source: Brown Wilson (2007).

Families also have important contributions to make to the community of the residential environment. This can range from having conversations with other residents who might not have visitors, helping staff by organising clothes or being involved in meals or afternoon tea rounds. Engaging in different activities brings families into contact with staff and so relationships are able to be developed. Families who engaged in these actions would demonstrate to me they had developed a shared understanding of what was happening in the home. For example, one son told me how he understood there were times when staff were busy, which meant his dad might have to wait for non-essential care. However, he also told me that when his dad did need care, staff would always provide this immediately. This understanding enabled negotiation between families and staff when views about what was needed for the resident differed. For families to reach this point, staff had to engage in person-centred care by demonstrating consistent attention to important details of care.

A person with dementia may not be able to engage in negotiation verbally when they need something different but changes in their behaviour may well be an indication that a change to the usual routine is needed at this point. Understanding this and acknowledging the feelings being communicated may well be part of the negotiation process as the staff or family member considers the impact this might have on the routines for the day ahead. Anticipating the difficulties this pressure might create for different people and attempting to consider the way in which the routines might be enacted in a different way may help satisify the needs of everyone in the relationship.

Conclusion

Returning to the concept of a continuum of care, we have seen that when viewed together individualised, person-centred and relationship-centred care can be viewed as a continuum where the everyday routines provide a vehicle to develop a greater understanding of the person with dementia, their family or significant other and staff. This might be best described as a cycle of care (see Figure 2.5).

Residents and families consider individualised care to be the minimum standard where choice is offered and likes and dislikes are recognised and acted upon. This

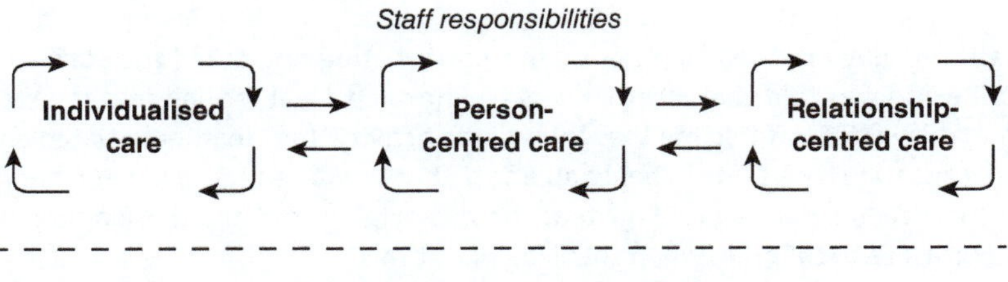

Figure 2.5 Continuum of care

could be considered a precursor for person-centred care, as the routines become a vehicle by which staff get to know the person with dementia and their family. This could be described as knowing 'what' is needed in the care routines. Sharing stories leads to an increased biographical knowledge that enables staff to understand why different routines are significant and how they underpin the personhood of the person with dementia. We might describe this as the 'why' of care as we understand the significance of the routines from the perspective of the person with dementia. Relationship-centred care maintains the importance of the personhood of the person with dementia (Nolan et al., 2004) but also means that the needs of families and staff can also be recognised alongside the needs of that person (Ryan et al., 2008). We could describe this as the 'how' of care as we recognise and value that everyone in the care relationship has a contribution to make, anticipate needs, develop shared understandings and be prepared to negotiate to ensure everyone's needs are met. To achieve this, a culture of community is required that enables shared understandings and negotiation (Brown Wilson and Davies, 2009; Brown Wilson, 2009). This is of particular relevance in communal environments where person-centred care is being enacted in a group context.

There is still limited empirical work on relationship-based approaches to care. This may be due to the difficulty in identifying relevant outcomes that are directly influenced by the process of care. This has been addressed to some degree in person-centred care as demonstrated by the good quality evidence reviewed in this chapter where we saw that agitation was directly influenced by person-centred approaches (Chenoweth et al., 2009, 2014). It was interesting to note that not all outcomes reached statistical significance and this may be due to other influences on the outcomes measured beyond the immediate impact of the care being delivered by staff. These may be issues beyond the control of staff in the wider organisation. In the next chapter, we will explore how the wider context of an organisation might impact on how relationship-based approaches to care might be implemented.

Final reflection

As people with dementia continue their journey, they will come into contact with services at times when they are less able to communicate what is important to them.

Our key responsibility as professionals in this field is to consider how to develop therapeutic relationships with the person with dementia, their families and significant others as well as the staff we work with. It is very easy to simply stay at the individualised care end of the continuum and believe we are implementing person-centred care. Unless we understand the importance of biography and what this means for the person with dementia, we will not be delivering person-centred care. We will revisit the key principles from this chapter as we journey through this book.

Further reading

Books

Brooker, D. and Latham, I. (2015) *Person-Centred Dementia Care: Making Services Better with the VIPS Framework* (second edition). Jessica Kingsley Publishers.

Brown Wilson, C. (2013) *Caring for Older People: A Shared Approach.* London: Sage Publications.

Websites

Christine Bryden is a dementia survivor and advocate. This website provides an insight into Christine's journey and experience: www.christinebryden.com/ (accessed 26/01/17).

The VIPS website has resources to support organisations in implementing the VIPS model: www.carefitforvips.co.uk (accessed 26/01/17).

3

The role of the organisation in leading and facilitating relationship-based dementia care

Learning objectives

By the end of this chapter, the reader will be able to:

- Explain how a Complex Adaptive System could promote relationship-based dementia care.
- Examine the components of a Complex Adaptive System at all levels of an organisation.
- Identify how the components of a Complex Adaptive System act as a facilitator or barrier for delivering relationship-based dementia care.
- Evaluate how working with staff in a Complex Adaptive System will enable the development of relationship-based approaches to care in the organisation.

Introduction

Healthcare organisations are often hierarchical, rule bound and can be slow to embrace innovation and change. Such inflexibility creates a focus on the task and limits creativity as staff feel they may be censured for not strictly adhering to the rules of the system. However, many healthcare organisations now espouse patient- or person-centred philosophies and consequently staff focusing on the task may seem out of step with the values of the organisation in which they work. On the other hand, staff feel they need to focus on the task in order to achieve the immediate outcomes expected by the institution. Many of these outcomes are focused on patient safety and quality of care and as such seek to reduce the incidence of problems such as falls, incontinence and pressure ulcers as examples. This in turn, creates a tension for staff who seek to implement person-centred care but are obliged to restrict their time to focusing on these measurable outcomes. Hierarchical rule-bound systems are equally challenging for students who are trying to learn different approaches to practice but feel constrained by the expectations of the institution in which they are practising. In the previous chapter, we found that the implementation of person-centred care practice had limited impact on outcomes for the person with dementia. This may be that the changes to practice were being implemented in organisations that were very rule bound and provided limited flexibility for staff to practise in different ways. Organisations that depend on a hierarchical structure with a focus on rules to manage behaviour of workers, can be likened to 'machines' where there is a belief that a change in one area of the machine is likely to have a predictable effect on another part of the machine. Lyn Chenoweth's CADRES study demonstrates that a change in practice may have unpredictable effects on outcomes, such as increasing the amount of falls (Chenoweth et al., 2009). This chapter seeks to explain unpredictable outcomes by using an alternative mental model of the organisation as a Complex Adaptive System. We will consider how using this organisational model may bridge the gap between an organisation's stated mission and values and the day-to-day practice of staff. This chapter proposes that dementia care needs organisations that can adapt in meeting the needs of the person with dementia and their families. We will consider the definition and components of organisations as Complex Adaptive Systems and then the actions required at each level of the organisation to achieve relationship-based approaches to care. As a student or novice practitioner, you might be focused on the *micro*, that is the local level of care delivery, but as you progress in your career and begin to lead teams you will be influencing the *meso*, or middle level of an organisation. Senior managers influence the *macro* or broader level of the organisation, which in turn dictates how care is delivered at both the meso and micro level of an organisation. This chapter will demonstrate how each level of an organisation is connected and how these connections influence care delivery. Adopting an organisational perspective is the first step in leading and managing change to improve outcomes for people living with dementia within the organisation in which we practise. Change can be effected at any level of the organisation but will be most effective when the change is represented at each of the *macro*, *meso* and *micro* levels.

Organisations as Complex Adaptive Systems

Complexity theory is a collection of theories that have emerged to explain why some systems show patterns of adaptability in response to an ever-changing environment. Complexity science is considered a successor to systems theory where linear processes were thought to result in specific outcomes such as in the 'machine metaphor' described in the introduction (Chaffee and McNeill, 2007). Complexity theory focuses on Complex Adaptive Systems (CAS) to describe patterns of behaviour in social systems, economies, cultures and organisations where behaviour does not appear to occur in a linear fashion (Dooley, 1997). Complex patterns have been investigated in seemingly random data such as in beehives, shoals of fish or flocks of birds. The pattern of behaviour demonstrated that the whole was more than the sum of its parts with a network of information passing through the shoal or flock so that every individual adjusts its behaviour in exactly the correct way to ensure the whole stays intact whilst it moves direction or is responsive to an external threat. This theory has also been applied to organisations, taking over the machine metaphor where there was a linear hierarchy where all parts had specific functions, with limited or no interaction with other parts of the organisation (see Table 3.1, after Dooley, 1997).

Table 3.1 Comparison between organisations as CAS and machines after Dooley, 1997

Defining features of an organisation as a Complex Adaptive System	Defining features of an organisation as a machine
Order emerges as new information becomes available and can be actioned at any part of the organisation	Order is pre-determined by the organisational structure with the head making decisions and the workers carrying them out
The building blocks of a CAS are agents; these may be staff or others who come into contact with the organisation	The hierarchy of the organisation determines the change. External people are only able to influence through the control that the hierarchy has within the organisation
Agents (such as employees) scan their environment both internally (other agents) and externally to develop cognitive schema, which define how they interact with other agents	Workers are kept in specific units and not encouraged to interact with others outside of formal processes
Change is dynamic and unpredictable; what happens in one part of the organisation will impact on another part of the organisation	Change is predictable and where it has effect will be determined by the linear nature of the organisation
Tags facilitate the formation of sub units within an organisation that facilitate change by their interactions	Sub units are determined by the hierarchy and do not always have links with other units

Globalisation and the changing financial landscape have caused theorists to rethink organisational theory to enable organisations to be more responsive in a constantly changing environment (Dooley, 1997). The theoretical perspective of Complex Adaptive Systems has been applied to healthcare systems as a mechanism to improve innovation and outcomes for people receiving care (McDaniel and Driebe, 2001; Anderson et al., 2003; Rouse, 2008; Plsek, 2003; Stroebel et al., 2005).

Plsek and Greenhaulgh (2001: 625) provide a succinct definition of a Complex Adaptive System as:

> a collection of individual agents with freedom to act in ways that are not totally predictable and whose actions are interconnected so that one agent's actions change the context for other agents.

A Complex Adaptive System (CAS) has a number of properties that enable it to adapt (Table 3.2). A key feature relevant to dementia care is self-organisation, where people mutually adjust their behaviours to cope with internal or external demands, that has an unpredictable impact on the organisation and would not have been possible without the variety of agents involved (Cilliers, 1998). For example, a person with dementia might not wish to get out of bed at the time that a staff member approaches them. This means the staff member has to adapt their routine and may need to negotiate this with other members of staff, so creating a different routine for that shift. This self-adaptive behaviour means that the organisation is capable of learning and so evolving (Dooley, 1997; Plsek and Greenhaulgh, 2001). The underpinning rationale

Table 3.2 Properties of Complex adaptive Systems (adapted from Plsek and Greenhaulgh, 2001, McDaniel and Driebe, 2001, Anderson et al, 2003, Chaffee and McNeill, 2007)

Property of a CAS	Description of property	How this might look in a dementia care organisation
Relationships between agents	Interaction between agents creates behaviour patterns within an organisation that produces new and unpredictable possibilities that would not have emerged by agents acting alone. The whole becomes more than the sum of its parts.	Staff, people with dementia receiving care and their families are all agents within a dementia care environment. Regulatory authorities could also be considered as agents.
Adaptation	Agents and the system are adaptive through interactions between agents and the wider environment which results in learning and different ways of behaving.	Relationship-based approaches to care that include the contribution of people with dementia and families encourage interaction between agents and provide information that can be used by staff to be flexible in approaching their care.
Co-evolution	Systems are embedded within other systems and co-evolve as tensions and balance change in either the internal or external environment influencing the interaction of agents. Each agent and system is nested within each other and influences each other.	Staff are agents on a dementia unit which is an agent in the CAS of a larger organisation such as a hospital or nursing home. The regulatory system influences the CAS of the larger organisation, which then influences the interaction between agents in the unit.

(Continued)

Table 3.2 (Continued)

Property of a CAS	Description of property	How this might look in a dementia care organisation
Emergence	Interaction leads to emerging novel behaviour as a result of co-evolution. Sudden and unpredicted phenomena emerge due to these interactions and within the CAS.	Relationships are integral to the functioning of a dementia unit and leaders focus on the development of positive relationships between all agents.
Self-organisation	Interactions within a CAS can create both order and innovation by following simple shared rules of behaviour that may be internalised and described as a 'mental model' such as 'do unto others'.	If person-centred care does not fit in with staff mental models it may be difficult to implement changes to care practice. Mental models may be apparent in the motivations staff describe when working in dementia care. Understanding staff motivation is the first step in understanding how staff self-organise.
Non-linearity	There is no fixed result from an action – one action may result in a number of different responses. A small change may have a larger than expected impact and a large change may have no impact.	Changing the meal times on one unit may have an impact on the preparation of meals across the organisation and the time of meals for other clients in the organisation.
Unpredictability	It is not possible to predict the pattern of a CAS as there is no fixed result from any one action.	Implementing person-centred care for one person may mean that another person's care may need to alter, having an impact on that person which may not be predictable.
Attractors	Having similar values may cause agents to attract within a system and so exert influence in the CAS.	A protocol for person-centred care could act as an attractor between staff who wish to implement a change in practice.
Cognitive diversity	The more agents involved in the decision making means there are more ways of thinking about a situation and so a better outcome may be generated.	Involving all workers responsible for direct care in considering an issue with a client may support an improved decision as many perspectives may support a more appropriate outcome.

for this evolution is that when an organisation is pushed from its usual state of equilibrium it can spontaneously organise into new structures responding quickly to internal or external stimuli (McDaniel and Driebe, 2001). In our example, the internal stimulus was in respecting the perspective of the person with dementia in not wanting to get out of bed at a pre-arranged time. However, self-organisation cannot be controlled in that it can only be influenced by shared values and purpose (Dooley, 1997).

In our example, the values are those of person-centred care that influence the relationships developed with other staff as well as the person with dementia. Relationships are central to a Complex Adaptive System as they influence the interactions between people (or agents) and the interconnections these people have with each other as well as the organisational or wider environment. The more diversity within the interactions and the more 'agents' involved, the greater the opportunity for new thinking to emerge and more creative ways of working (Chaffee and McNeill, 2007). Just as we examined the importance of relationships in care delivery (Chapter 2), considering relationships from an organisational perspective will also enable us to examine how organisations might become dementia friendly.

Many people with dementia receive care in highly regulated institutions with formalised control, which reduces the need for interaction between staff, thus stifling innovation or creativity (Anderson et al., 2003). Table 3.2 considers dementia care environments as Complex Adaptive Systems (CAS) where agents within an organisation are connected via networks rather than linear relationships thus enabling improvisation and responsive ways of acting (Cilliers, 1998). Effective relationships between agents is central to CAS and how people relate to each other enables effective problem solving resulting in different ways of working (Jordan et al., 2010). The following sections explore how a CAS works at the different levels of an organisation starting at the micro level of the CAS where we enact direct care.

Agents and interactions within the system

Agents within an organisation could be defined as the people within the organisation as well as stakeholders such as those in receipt of services. Rouse (2008) speaking about the design of healthcare as a Complex Adaptive System suggests all stakeholders including competitor organisations, customers (clients or patients) and regulators should be taken into account.

Activity 3.1 Reflection

Who are the agents within your organisation?

Draw a network diagram that demonstrates the key agents. Start with the person with dementia, then chart the degrees of proximity regarding each of the following stakeholders: family and supporters, direct care staff, registered nursing staff, other healthcare professionals, managers, regulating authorities.

Put in arrows between the different groups to demonstrate the flow of information.

In a dementia-friendly organisation, the person with dementia, their family and supporters should be considered as key agents with their perspectives taken into account. Equally, staff who are closest to the care and support of the person with dementia have views and perspectives that will influence the implementation of person-centred or relationship-centred care. There will also be registered allied healthcare professionals such as nurses and medical professionals. Interactions between staff occur through conversations, which may simply be to exchange information. However, when a team wishes to collaborate this also occurs through conversations. Conversations are ways that people think together, problem solve and develop different ways of doing things. In this context, the diversity of perspectives encourages organisational learning as new practices are implemented (Jordan et al., 2009). Diverse agents relate to each other in different ways, which can be used to develop creative and innovative approaches to care that reflect the perspective of the person with dementia.

Conversations are also vehicles by which relationships are developed with older people, including those with dementia, and their families. Personal information may be shared during care routines and/or visits that contribute to personal knowledge developed by the staff who hear these stories (Brown Wilson, 2007). Biographical information is the cornerstone of person-centred and relationship-centred care but is rarely reflected in care planning documents. This may be due to the informality of these exchanges or the similarity to storytelling (Boal and Schultz, 2007). Communication openness is a key feature of a CAS, enabling agents within the organisation to have access to a variety of information, so prompting learning and subsequent innovation (Anderson et al., 2003). In the studies we reviewed in earlier chapters, communication of biographical information was a key feature in many of the person-centred interventions. For example, Brooker and Woolley (2007) describe a member of staff as the 'Locksmith' where the sharing of biographical information with direct care staff was seen as the key to unlocking the potential for person-centred care within the organisation. Similarly, Rokstad et al. (2013) used regular staff meetings to enable information about residents to be shared by direct care staff and the whole team then developed solutions. Conversely an observation made in the CADRES study suggested that the solutions in Dementia Care Mapping were more likely to come from the person doing the mapping whereas the person-centred care approach meant that there was more of a collective approach in developing strategies (Chenoweth et al., 2009). These examples demonstrate the use of cognitive diversity to come up with a collective solution rather than being dependent upon one person.

Activity 3.2 Reflection

Return to your diagram in Activity 3.1.

Using a different colour pen, and adjusting the thickness of the line, draw in how often the interactions occur between each of the groups in your diagram. When there are limited interactions, make this a dotted line (monthly). As the interactions become less often make this a very light dotted line. When there are regular interactions (such as weekly) make this a thin line, with daily interactions being a thick/bold line.

Consider the following:

- Who are the majority of interactions between – does this represent cognitive diversity?
- How often is the wider team involved in interactions – how might this be increased to increase cognitive diversity?
- Are there any groups that don't interact regularly – how might you encourage additional interaction to develop cognitive diversity?

Understanding how we interact and who we interact with is the first step in developing innovative strategies to improve the care and support for people living with dementia. Developing responsive relationships between staff, the person with dementia and their families enables the relationship-centred approaches examined in Chapter 2 to occur. Relationships also influence how self-organisation occurs within Complex Adaptive Systems.

Self-organisation

People self-organise to create new behaviours to meet the demands of the relationships they have with each other and their environment (McDaniel and Driebe, 2001). This statement resonates with the philosophy of relationship-based approaches to care, which are founded on personal and responsive relationships (Brown Wilson, et al., 2009). To this end, supporting direct care staff to make their own decisions in the organisation of care has the potential to promote self-organisation. For example, in my observations in residential aged care, staff who were responsive to resident needs and understood what was important to those residents in the routines of the home, were described as the 'A team' (Brown Wilson, 2007). When I spoke to members of this team, it became apparent they all had a similar motivation, 'to make a difference'. These motivations acted as attractors between different members of staff and explained why different teams of people worked well together.

Activity 3.3 Reflection

- Think of the reason why you chose nursing or healthcare as a profession.
- Write down the values you believe in as a professional.
- Write down the motivation you have in the care you deliver.
- What impact do you think these values and your motivation has on the person living with dementia and their families?
- What impact do you think these values and your motivation has on other staff?
- What is the evidence you have used to reach these conclusions?

In Chapter 2, we saw how individualised, person-centred and relationship-centred care were delivered by staff with differing motivations (Figure 2.5). When the motivation was to 'do a good job' then the attractor or focus of that team was individualised care (Brown Wilson and Davies, 2009). As individualised care was focusing on the task which followed a set routine, self-organisation was limited. When staff moved towards person-centred care, they described their motivation as 'Do unto others' – in that they provided the care that was important to the resident because that was how they would like care to be provided to them (Brown Wilson and Davies, 2009). The attractor for person-centred care was the focus on the person enabling a more flexible approach to be adopted in care delivery, which could be described as self-organisation. The staff who described their motivation as 'making a difference' demonstrated a greater level of responsiveness as they anticipated the needs of those they cared for and acted before problems emerged. Multiple perspectives were needed to achieve this level of self-organisation and these were gathered through informal conversations and information sharing across the shift.

Practice scenario 3.1

In my observations of relationship-centred care I observed staff interacting informally throughout the day as they passed throughout the care home, sharing anecdotes and stories about the residents. This included sharing biographical information that was relevant to the care for that day. Interactions occurred with all levels of staff including the nurse manager. If care needed to be altered due to a change of condition, decisions were made jointly and escalated in a responsive manner. This meant that staff would reorganise their care to suit the changing needs of different residents, taking into account the needs of all stakeholders. For residents who were more able, this might involve a re-negotiation of the usual care routine for that day. These residents felt part of the wider community and saw their cooperation with the proposed change as an opportunity to support less able residents. This self-organisation enabled person-centred care to be enacted for individual residents in the context of the wider community of the nursing home.

Source: from Brown Wilson (2007).

Practice scenario 3.1 demonstrates how staff engagement in regular and informal interaction enables a more adaptive response in a dynamic healthcare situation. Anderson et al. (2005a) suggest that diverse interactions produce a better understanding of a situation. In healthcare environments, there is a wealth of cognitive diversity with differing perspectives of staff, people with dementia and their families. Encouraging informal interaction within teams enables staff to develop shared understandings thus moving along the continuum to relationship-centred care (Figure 2.4). However, I also observed staff sharing anecdotes and stories related to their care during informal interactions. Sharing stories is often the way in which people make sense of the world and so helps in understanding the visible behaviour in an organisation (Boal and Schultz, 2007).

Leadership

So far we have considered the building blocks of a Complex Adaptive System at the level of direct care or the *micro* level of the organisation. However, to enable front-line staff to be responsive to the changing needs of residents and so facilitate person-centred care, an open and inclusive management style is needed (Brooker and Woolley, 2007). When staff feel supported with clear boundaries and expectations, they are more likely to take responsibility in the care they deliver (Killett et al., 2013). Management is generally aligned to the mid or *meso* level of the organisation with leadership at this level enabling or constraining the opportunities for self-organisation. For example, Anderson and McDaniel (1998) found that an overreliance on formal mechanisms gave Registered Nurses less influence in decision-making than more informal mechanisms. As many health and care organisations are highly regulated, some leaders or managers may feel it is more appropriate to ensure care is being delivered through prescriptive rules and routines, which may inadvertently perpetuate task-focused approaches.

Practice scenario 3.2

In the Beeches, the Nurse Manager led from the front by role modelling person-centred practice and supporting staff who might not be implementing this consistently. The Nurse Manager described this approach as explaining to staff 'how we do things around here', implying there were shared values across the home. This Nurse Manager was also visible during the delivery of care interacting informally with the staff as information was shared and all staff contributed to problem solving as issues emerged. When care plans were being written or updated, all staff involved in the care were involved. By contrast, in HolyOakes, the Nurse Manager primarily communicated via memos and was rarely visible during the care routines. She informed me that she had directed staff to be more person-centred but she still found staff were being assigned to tasks by the Team Leaders on each unit. Information was shared through team meetings at specified times and direct care staff informed me they were rarely involved in care planning meetings.

Source: based on Brown Wilson (2009).

We can see from Practice scenario 3.2 that differing leadership styles may act as a facilitator or barrier to self-organisation. For example, adopting a hierarchical model alone will not prevent self-organisation, but simply starve it of the interconnections and cognitive diversity needed to make decisions (Anderson et al., 2003). Brooker and Woolley (2007) contend that specialist expertise in dementia is a key component of implementing a sustainable model of person-centred care. In this Enriched Opportunities Programme (EOP) the leadership provided by the position of 'Locksmith' encouraged participation in decision-making and enabled decisions that might not be possible when less people are involved in decision-making. For example, Anderson and colleagues (2003) suggest that encouraging participation in decision-making when caring for people with dementia results in lower prevalence of aggressive and disruptive behaviours. Involving more perspectives in the decision-making process contributes to shared understandings promoting relationship-centred care (Brown Wilson, 2009).

The culture of the organisation

The mission and vision of an organisation is often decided at the macro level of the organisation and represents what the organisation stands for. Organisational statements are important and provide guidance to staff contributing in part to shared values (Killett et al., 2013). Many organisations now include the principles of person-centred care in their mission and vision for the organisation, with many dementia care organisations developing their own model. PEARL (Positively Enriching And enhancing Residents Lives; Baker, 2015) is an example of a programme developed by a for-profit care organisation in the UK that has developed person-centered care into a form of accreditation across their network of residential dementia care environments. This includes guidance and training for staff in how to implement these principles in everyday care routines (Baker, 2015). However the culture of an organisation is more than a mission statement. Culture is built on implicit assumptions and values (Doll, 2003), which may be shared and developed through the informal interactions we have explored in earlier sections of this chapter. Informal interactions connect people with dementia and their families with staff, thus developing a sense of community (Brown Wilson, 2009; Killett et al., 2013). Active sharing of biographical stories certainly contributes to staff implementing person-centred daily care routines (Brown Wilson and Davies, 2009). Regular and informal interactions also contribute to the sense of the 'way we do things around here' that actively influences the culture of the organisation (Brown Wilson, 2009).

Activity 3.4 Reflection

In the organisation in which you are practising, find a copy of a mission statement. If there is no mission statement available, ask staff how they would describe the mission of the organisation.

- Compare these mission statements with the values you identified in Activity 3.3.
- How are these similar or different?
- How does this influence your judgement about this organisation?

We know that staff will experience greater levels of satisfaction if the organisational values align with their own (Bell, 2014). This congruence between the organisational and personal values will influence the type of stories people share within an organisation. These stories contribute to a mental representation of that organisation that is communicated and shared with others (Boal and Schultz, 2007). A system of open communication and interaction, facilitated in a CAS generates new knowledge (Anderson et al., 2003) that enables the organisation to develop a life story of its own (Boal and Schultz, 2007). Studies by Ruth Anderson and colleagues, discussed in the previous section, suggest that increased participation in decision-making improves outcomes for both staff and people with dementia (Anderson et al., 2003). However, some staff may need support in how to participate effectively in decision-making and to change the way they practice.

The mission statement of an organisation should also include how they intend to support the staff in being able to implement the mission of the organisation. Training staff in the principles of care required by the organisation is often a logical first step. However, a belief that training staff will automatically result in changed behaviour favours the organisation as a machine metaphor. The premise goes that if we train staff in the correct way of providing person-centred care, this means they will automatically deliver this. If they don't, then there must be something wrong with the staff such as educational attainment, problems with language or communication, attitude etc. Staff, however, need support in how to adopt different practices such as communicating with people with dementia and staff training is often seen as lacking particularly in the care home sector (Killett et al., 2013).

If we consider dementia care environments as CAS, then we also need to consider a model of knowledge transfer that is relevant to promoting self-organisation and including cognitive diversity. In a small-scale study involving two care homes, myself and colleagues used the Senses Framework (Table 2.1) as a mechanism to support staff in caring for people living with dementia to view their care differently (Brown Wilson et al., 2013). These staff had been trained in person-centred care but were having difficulty in implementing the principles in everyday practice. We utilised a process of Practice Development supporting staff to apply evidence to their practice, influencing knowledge, attitudes and actions of staff (McCormack, 2011). Practice Development includes a deliberate aim of empowering staff to change practice though facilitation (Manley and McCormack, 2004). The focus of this approach is on supporting staff to critically reflect on their practice, identifying their own solutions using evidence from the literature. Support was provided to staff by a process of facilitation, where prompts were used to encourage staff to think of different ways of implementing the Senses Framework. For example, staff were encouraged to think about their own life and significant events that occurred and then to speak to a person with dementia and their family caregiver about significant events in their lives. This discussion prompted staff to initiate conversations with the person with dementia and their families. The information was then shared with other staff resulting in the emergence of novel ways to enact the care routines. The staff who were involved in this project came from different units across the home, which increased the cognitive diversity of the group. When one group implemented an idea in their unit, they would return the following week where the whole group would then discuss how to adapt the practice to other units, often creating new and diverse ways of implementing relationship-centred care. These sessions did not 'tell' people how to change their practice but enabled staff to identify how they could do things differently. Facilitation was fundamental to this process and gave the staff the opportunity to act on local wisdom (Anderson et al., 2005b) as the following practice scenario suggests.

Practice scenario 3.3

Staff were discussing how important music was to each of them and what music might mean for the person with dementia. Concerns were raised due to the lack of time in being able to develop activities for the residents. The following week staff told me how they had got talking to some of the people with dementia who told them how they had met their husbands or wives at 'dance halls'. This prompted staff to find some 'dance hall music' which they played one morning. Staff decided that rather than sitting in the office to write care plans, they would relocate to the lounge where they could also facilitate the music session. This resulted in an impromptu music session between morning tea and lunch time. Staff recounted how people who rarely communicated were tapping their feet or hands in time to the music with some residents spontaneously dancing together.

Source: reflections from Brown Wilson et al. (2013).

Practice scenario 3.3 provides an example of self-organisation based on diverse interactions involving a number of agents, on this occasion, the people with dementia and the staff in one unit. Ideas had been generated and strategies developed by staff who were responsible for implementing them. This meant that the solutions were able to be adapted into everyday routines, rather than being seen as additional workload. This is a very different approach to the didactic method of giving staff knowledge out of context and then expecting them to implement it during busy care routines. Practice scenario 3.3 is an example of how an organisation was able to support staff in implementing the mission and values of person-centred care.

Conclusion

A Complex Adaptive System is more than the sum of its parts. Informal and frequent interactions between those that work within the organisation enable new patterns of behaviour to emerge. This occurs by involving people with dementia, families and all levels of staff incorporating diverse perspectives into the interaction. Common forms of communication are the sharing of stories and conversations where people work together to problem solve. This enables staff to adapt their practice in a responsive way of working referred to as self-organisation. Examples from practice demonstrate how informally sharing stories and anecdotes is a powerful mechanism to support staff in implementing person-centred and relationship-centred care. Enabling the person with dementia and family members to participate in the decision-making process also has the potential to create new ways of working that includes all perspectives. Supporting staff to move along the continuum of care requires leadership and a facilitative approach to staff training. We will return to each of these in more detail in subsequent chapters.

Final reflections

In this chapter we have started a journey considering how we might implement the principles of relationship-based approaches to care into the real world of practice in healthcare organisations. To achieve this, we have used organisational theory to look at the micro, meso and macro levels of the organisations in which we practice. The following chapters will now apply this to everyday practice enabling us to consider what is needed at each level of an organisation to implement relationship-based dementia care.

Further reading

Leadership resources

Schein, E. (2010) *Organisational Culture and Leadership* (fourth edition). Josey Bass. Available at: www.ehs-club.com/Files/linli_mary/file/20150211/20150211124427_6412.pdf (accessed 10/09/16).

4

Developing a biographical approach in care practice

Learning objectives

By the end of this chapter, the reader will be able to:

- Examine how to implement a relationship-based model of dementia care by using a biographical approach to care planning.
- Explore how direct care is influenced by the structure of the organisation and how a Complex Adaptive System supports dementia care.
- Analyse the barriers and enablers at the care delivery level of the organisation that might impede or promote relationship-based approaches to care.
- Complete a care plan for a relationship-based model of dementia care.

Introduction

As we discussed in Chapter 2, valuing personhood is a fundamental principle of person-centred and relationship-centred care. We examined the value of biography in developing knowledge of what mattered to people living with dementia in everyday care routines. Understanding the person with dementia is the first stage in this process. This chapter will support you in adopting a biographical approach to care planning through your interactions with the person with dementia, their families and staff you work with. We will also explore how an organisational structure impacts on care delivery by influencing the diversity and amount of interactions that occur in daily routines. We return to the notion of organisations as Complex Adaptive Systems and explore how this theoretical lens might help to implement relationship-based approaches to care. Strategies used by students and practitioners in developing biographical knowledge of the person with dementia illustrate how positive outcomes can be facilitated. These strategies when considered as part of the broader organisational context are the first step in moving towards a dementia-friendly environment.

Understanding the person

Interactions during care routines provide a legitimate focus for families, people with dementia and staff (Brown Wilson et al., 2009; Clissett et al., 2013a) and are a useful starting point for the development of positive relationships (Brown Wilson et al., 2009). When positive relationships exist, there tend to be more opportunities for sharing information through care interactions. Equally, it is through the care interactions that relationships develop. These may be pragmatic (Brown Wilson et al., 2009), focusing primarily on the task. However, the cyclical nature of caregiving over time enables staff to develop knowledge about the person in how they react to different routines, how they engage with these routines and the type of person they are. Over time, this information may be augmented by stories shared by the person with dementia aided by personal artefacts about their life that could be a source of discussion, or by stories shared by families and friends. As this biographical knowledge develops, staff progress from pragmatic to personal and responsive relationships (Brown Wilson et al., 2009). It is at this point of using biographical knowledge to personalise care routines in ways that are meaningful for the person that person-centred care develops (Brown Wilson, 2012). There are reports that staff sometimes may adopt a more person-centred rhetoric, using this to frame current care, but without changing the way they do things (Doll, 2003). By framing person-centred care in relation to the way care is delivered, we provide a clearer framework for staff to understand the difference between undertaking a task-directed approach as compared to a person-centred approach.

All models of person-centred care talk about the importance of biography and knowing the person – this is not unique and most staff caring for people living with dementia would say they develop personal relationships with those they care for. In my observations of staff implementing a person-centred approach, the difference was in how they used this personal knowledge to influence the care they delivered and then how this was shared amongst the team, becoming the usual pattern of care delivery for that person (Brown Wilson, 2012). However, this information was rarely recorded in the assessment and care plan for the person. This meant that person-centred care was generally reliant on a single person or a group of people working together. The following section considers how we might move to a more consistent approach to ensure person-centred care becomes the norm across shifts irrespective of who is on duty.

Most of the literature related to biography focuses on the life story of an individual. Boal and Schultz (2007) suggest that an individual recalls elements of their life story in different ways to create an overall mental representation of their life and this structures the important events into a coherent autobiographical pattern meaningful to that person. Life review and life story books have been found to have a positive impact on the quality of life for people living with dementia in care homes. Life story books enable staff to understand the person and improve the relationship between the person with dementia and their families (Subramaniam et al., 2014). Implementing life review to create a life story book is a skilled process and is often beyond the time frame that staff have in their working day (Subramaniam et al., 2014). Indeed, when biographical information is not available to staff, behaviours of people with dementia may be misinterpreted as challenging, becoming a source of frustration for staff. In Practice scenario 2.3 we explored the relevance of biographical information for Mr Au's behaviour. Staff had been able to contextualise Mr Au's behaviours in relation to his life story, which then prompted responses that supported the wellbeing of Mr Au. To ensure Mr Au's ongoing wellbeing, staff needed to work together to consistently implement this approach.

Putting people who work well together seems to make very good sense but often there is little consideration as to why different people work well together. In Chapter 2 we saw that the personal motivation of staff was a key influence on the approach to care being adopted. The personal motivation of staff can also affect relationships within teams. When people identify similar philosophies then they are more likely to accept suggestions to work more flexibly recognising the different skills amongst the team (Brown Wilson, 2009). Equally, conflicting philosophies of care may result in friction with each member of the team believing their way is the best way. Not all members of the team necessarily start off with the same philosophy but as they recognise the impact of different care styles on the wellbeing of the resident, they adapt their behaviour to experience improved care interactions. Practice scenario 4.1 demonstrates how the philosophy of teams may influence individual members.

Practice scenario 4.1

A young staff member was working as a care assistant whilst waiting to train as a healthcare professional. She started off with a very pragmatic approach, wanting to do a good job. She was working with a team that espoused and enacted a person-centred philosophy in everyday care interactions. Over a three-month period, this staff member began describing her care in personal and responsive terms that mirrored other members of the team. When I asked her about her changed approach, she explained that adopting a person-centred approach resulted in improved care interactions for her, the person with dementia and the family members.

Source: from Brown Wilson (2007), unpublished data.

From the example above, the staff in this team espoused a personal philosophy that motivated them to adopt person-centred practice and encouraged newer members of the team to adopt similar practices (Brown Wilson, 2007). The level of flexibility and self-organisation occurring in direct care delivery may also be influenced by the personal philosophy of staff. Staff who implemented person-centred or relationship-centred care in my research described different motivations that brought them into a caring role (Brown Wilson, 2012). It is often difficult to recruit and retain good quality staff in the care sector. I worked with one organisation to develop person-centred role descriptions that reflected the vision and philosophy of the service and these positions were filled in a geographical area that had been traditionally difficult to recruit from.

Activity 4.1 Critical thinking

As a Registered Nurse (RN) in training, how would you describe your values and demonstrate how you implement them in everyday care? **Avoid** using the words person-centred or relationship-centred and focus on what you mean by these concepts and what you might do to demonstrate these concepts.

Role	Values	Experience to demonstrate these values
Registered Nurse		

Staff who wished to make a difference in the lives of those they cared for were often found to be implementing relationship-centred care (Figure 2.4) by juggling competing care demands to ensure everyone received the attention to detail that was important to those they cared for (Brown Wilson, 2012). This level of biographical knowledge contributed to the ability to anticipate what was needed before it became an issue which meant person-centred care was being delivered in spite of what might have been considered to be competing priorities. This occurred through a process of negotiation and compromise, made possible by spontaneous conversations (Brown Wilson, 2012). Conversations between staff are an emergent pattern within a Complex Adaptive System: as conversations are jointly constructed, new meanings emerge and individuals improvise on a situation using both rules and adaptation as they make decisions in the moment (Jordan et al., 2009). The meanings that emerged from these conversations and subsequent decisions developed into shared understandings about the people being cared for and the way that care needed to be delivered. For those staff who valued relationships, conversations between staff were usually focused on what was important for the person with dementia and would generally draw on biographical knowledge (Brown Wilson et al., 2009).

Developing shared understandings though diverse interactions

Within residential aged care, conversations frequently occur between staff, staff and residents, staff and families, between residents and between residents and families, creating a diversity of interaction that leads to a sense of community. Recognising and valuing the contribution older people and families make to the life and community of the home is an integral part of relationship-based approaches to care (Brown Wilson et al., 2009). In my work and research in care homes, I often observed residents helping others – for example, one woman would sit next to another who had difficulty in hearing so she could let her know what was going on in the home (Brown Wilson et al., 2009). Another gentleman used to always deliver the post around the home and he would spend time chatting with many of the other residents. In subsequent studies people with dementia describe similar patterns of behaviour in providing comfort to others or helping out around the home when they can (Moyle et al., 2013b). Family members also described how they found ways of being involved in the home, giving them a sense they were contributing to the community of the home by helping staff where needed (Brown Wilson et al., 2009). Although this varied according to the families involved and therefore was not static, when staff became aware of the contribution family members made to the home's community, development of reciprocal relationships occurred (Brown Wilson et al., 2009). These reciprocal relationships contributed to families describing shared understandings when they could see how staff managed competing priorities (Brown Wilson and Davies, 2009). This was in direct contrast with studies that report antagonistic relationships between family members and staff, with staff seeing families as a distraction rather than making a contribution (Hertzberg et al., 2003; Bauer, 2006; Utley-Smith et al., 2009).

Creating opportunities for interactions between staff, residents and families has been shown to promote the exchange of information, which can be applied by staff to promote wellbeing by making a difference in the care of the residents (Bauer, 2006; Brown Wilson et al., 2009; Utley-Smith et al., 2009). Soderstrom et al. (2003), in a study in intensive care units, suggest staff use two types of behaviours towards families: inviting and non-inviting. When staff used inviting behaviours, this led to a greater sense of trust with families who then felt able to spend less time on the unit as demonstrated in Practice scenario 4.2.

Practice scenario 4.2

Flo would always come and see the staff on duty. She would ask them about her husband, Ernie and share anecdotes with them about their lives together. The team leader told me that she would always make time for Flo as this was an opportunity to learn more about Ernie. It also meant that Flo felt connected with Ernie's care. Flo told me that she now felt able to take one day away from the home where she would go to a carers' support meeting because she felt more comfortable with the staff knowing they were caring for her husband.

When provided with opportunities to do so, families seek interaction with staff (Utley-Smith et al., 2009) and it is the focus of these interactions that shapes the type of relationship developed. For example, in the studies I have undertaken, when staff recognised the significance of biographical knowledge, this provided opportunities for social exchange with families and the person with dementia as described in the above scenario. These conversations then supported residents and families in making an active contribution towards the development of personal and responsive or reciprocal relationships with staff (Brown Wilson et al., 2009). As shared understandings develop, the needs of all stakeholders within the relationship are acknowledged: the person in receipt of care, families and staff, which then contributes towards a sense of community within the home (Brown Wilson, 2009; Killett et al., 2016).

Activity 4.2 Take action

Use the following checklist (based on the work of Utley-Smith et al., 2009) to assess the interaction with families in the organisation in which you practise.

Activity	Always	Sometimes	Rarely	Never
Staff actively seek out the family to share information when they visit				
Staff communicate about the person's condition without family having to request information				
Staff use the telephone or written information to inform family members if something different happens in the person's care				
Staff express an interest in family's wellbeing				
Staff provide explanations for treatment in a non-threatening manner				
Staff engage families in care planning				
Family meetings are held regularly				

Action plan

Identify the actions that could be taken to increase the interaction between staff and families in the organisation in which you practise:

Formal activity	Informal activity

Using biographical information in assessment and care planning

In the previous sections, we have discussed how informal and frequent interactions between staff and with families enable flexible responses to residents' needs thus promoting self-organisation as all levels of staff engage in care-related decision-making (Anderson et al., 2005a, 2013). This section will focus on how the shared understandings that emerge from these diverse interactions go on to shape the care interactions involving the person with dementia. Many conversations and interactions will emerge from an individual care interaction and are shared with others through conversation, which then create a new meaning and subsequent shared understanding. Our understanding of organisations as Complex Adaptive Systems suggest this shared understanding can be used in the care interaction enabling the staff member to engage in new behaviours thus delivering a different approach to care (see Figure 4.1). It is at this point that the staff member is moving along the continuum towards person-centred care as they acknowledge the biography of the person in the care routines they deliver.

Often I hear staff sharing important biographical information to help other staff understand the behaviour of a person with dementia. However, it is rare that this information is written down or included as part of the handover of care for that person. In the previous chapters we read about the Enriching Opportunities Programme that identified a 'Locksmith' who was assigned responsibility for undertaking a biographical assessment, sharing this with the direct care staff and then role modelling good practice (Brooker and Woolley, 2007). Other care environments might have a 'keyworker' or 'primary nurse' system, similar to the 'Locksmith' who is responsible for getting to know a group of people and completing their care records and other duties as specified by the unit they are working in.

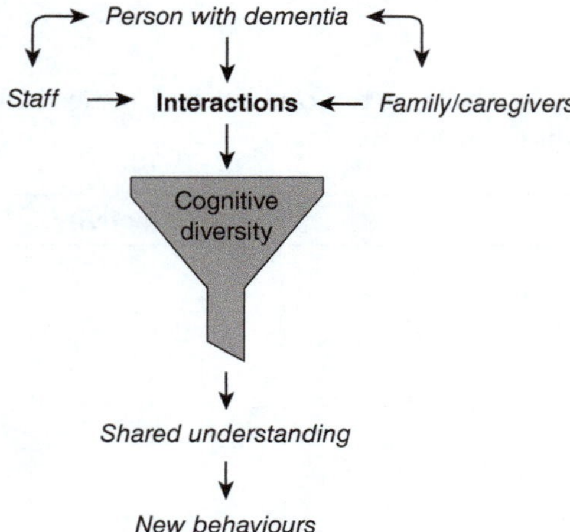

Figure 4.1 Process of developing shared understandings

However, this might be dependent upon what the assigned individual member of staff sees as important whereas a programme such as the EOP identifies very clear information requirements, ensuring important biographical information is included, with responsibility to demonstrate how to implement the information. Whilst many staff might agree this information is relevant they might not necessarily know how to implement it or feel they have the power to make the decision to do so. Other staff may believe that in recognising biographical information, they are delivering person-centred care. Supporting staff to understand how this information can be used within care routines is the first step in moving from individualised task-centred care to person-centred care. For example, engaging the person with dementia in meaningful activity that respects their ability to make decisions and remain involved in the world around them is central to a number of models of person-centred dementia care (Brooker and Woolley, 2007; Chenoweth et al., 2014; Moyle et al., 2016).

Wendy Moyle and colleagues (2016) developed the Capabilities Model of Dementia Care (CMDC) adopting a person-centred, relationship-centred and strengths-based approach focusing on the capabilities of the person with dementia rather than the deficiencies of the condition. The underpinning philosophy of this model is that the person with dementia's wellbeing is based on the opportunities to be the person they wish to be and engage in meaningful activities that enable them to achieve this. The aims of this model are to promote quality of life for the person with dementia, improve the experience of family members and improve the attitudes and experience of staff. CMDC follows a care cycle that: undertakes a multi-sources assessment; plans opportunities; facilitates care needs; and undertakes a case review and evaluation to enable the cycle to continue (Moyle et al., 2016). Unlike other models in dementia care, CMDC also includes a staffing component to ensure the correct amount and skills of staff exist to deliver the model (Moyle et al., 2016). Following implementation of this CMDC, residents with dementia expressed a positive view about the care they received, describing positive relationships with staff (Moyle et al., 2013b). Equally, staff reported how they believed they had been implementing person-centred care, but were able to recognise following the training that they had been focused on the task (Moyle et al., 2013b). This was underpinned by family observations of improved staff interactions where staff engaged with the person with dementia on a deeper level (Moyle et al., 2013b). Staff recognising that social exchange is an essential part of the daily routine with a person with dementia enables staff to see beyond the task to the person, contributing to reciprocal relationships (Brown Wilson and Davies, 2009; Killett et al., 2016). Including a biographical element to assessment and care planning ensures these important aspects of daily living are included.

Alzheimer's Associations internationally have developed resources to support people with dementia, families and staff in identifying significant biographical information. In the UK, 'This is me' is a document that has been developed for people living with dementia and their caregivers to take with them when moving between health and social care environments. 'This is me' enables staff at a glance to see important information about the activities of daily living and familiar routines which, should they be discontinued or go unsupported, may cause unnecessary distress to the person living with dementia.

In long-term residential care environments, it is useful to have a similar document that reflects meaningful activity to begin to frame this information in ways that staff can use. This is something that staff and families can work on together, promoting positive relationships from the beginning of the relationship. In this case, it is always a good idea to work with staff to identify the relevant questions to ask, so they engage with the process. An example of these questions is shown in Table 4.1.

Sharing biographical information as part of the usual record keeping of an organisation is always a challenge and finding out from staff how they use the records is the first step in ensuring direct care staff have access to important information that can shape the care routines. One group of staff I worked with in the UK explained they did not have time to look at the central records for each person they cared for and so developed a four-page booklet of photos and key phrases that was then laminated and located in the person's room (Brown Wilson et al., 2013). This was then used as a ready reference for all staff who engaged in the personal care of the person. Each member of staff constructed a booklet for one person and at the end of the project, each member of staff reported they knew more about the person with dementia and

Table 4.1 Understanding who I am

Where I have lived
The important people in my life
Pets I have shared my life with
Important dates in my life and why
Experiences I have had in my life
The good times and the smells that might remind me of these
Food that I enjoy
Food I really don't want to eat
The not so good times that I don't want to be reminded about
My achievements
Activities I enjoy
Activities I am good at
Things that irritate me and why
Music I enjoy and what it reminds me of
Films I have enjoyed in my life
What really matters to me
Important objects that remind me of what is important to me
What is important in my personal care routines
What makes me feel safe
What makes me feel unsafe
I would like to feel part of the community by:

were able to have meaningful conversations with them (Brown Wilson et al., 2013). This project used regular lunchtime meetings for staff from each unit to come together and look at ways of implementing relationship-centred care. By the end of the project, there was little facilitation required as staff themselves were identifying what was important and guiding the discussions. Providing staff with the time to consider and identify strategies that fit into their usual pattern of working was an effective way of implementing relationship-centred care on this occasion. This project succeeded in reframing the focus of staff, so it became about the person, rather than the task being undertaken; in this case, the personal care routines.

Wendy Moyle's Capability Model of Dementia Care (CMDC) demonstrated how staff were able to move from a task focus to a more person-centred approach (Moyle et al., 2013b). If we return to the notion of providing care along a continuum (Figure 2.5) staff could be described as moving along the continuum to seeing the person rather than the task. The CMDC encouraged staff to adapt their care thus matching the capabilities of the person with dementia and developing the care plan around ten capabilities enabling staff to maintain the capability focus (Moyle et al., 2016). This addresses some of the limitations of previous studies where person-centred care had not been documented (Chenoweth et al., 2014). Moyle et al. (2016) demonstrate how documentation within an organisation also needs to reflect the underpinning philosophy of the approach to care. The next step is now to integrate this information into the established care planning record systems within the organisation.

Activity 4.3 Critical thinking

Using life stories to develop care plans

- Choose one client with dementia that you know and support.
- Write down what you know about this person from conversations you have with them; include information from stories that have been shared with you.

Step 1: Knowing what is important to the person

- Identify personal routines they have had in the past – how is their life different now?
- Identify activities they might have done that gave them pleasure or their life meaning – who were these activities with? What does this tell you about this person?
- Do you see this person any differently now you know this information?

Step 2: Attention to details

- What are the important details for this person's care from what you know about this person?
- How might you include this information in this person's care?
- What meaningful activity might be important in the daily routines of this person?

(Continued)

(Continued)

Step 3: Consistent approach to care through record keeping

- How might you write this information in the care plan?
- How else might you communicate this information to everyone who supports this person?
- When a person with dementia tells you something about their life, how might you communicate this to the rest of the team?

Step 4: Valuing everyone's contribution

- What might you do if the family tells you something about this person that you don't know?
- How might you communicate this new information?
- What will it communicate to the family if you show you are using this information?
- Compare what you have written to the usual care plan – what are the key differences?
- How might you incorporate this information into your organisation's care plan?

Conclusion

This chapter has examined the key elements of direct care delivery in promoting relationship-based approaches to care. Focusing on the person with dementia, biography is an essential aspect of care planning if person-centred care is to be realised at the micro level of the organisation. The enabling features of a Complex Adaptive System include the personal motivation of staff, and the diversity of interaction to include staff, families and the person with dementia. Increasing this interaction allows an informal flow of communication that enhances the understanding of the person with dementia and promotes a flexible approach to care delivery. The final section of this chapter emphasises the value of integrating biographical knowledge into the formal care planning process thus ensuring a more person-centred focus in care delivery. In the following chapter, we will explore the role of the Registered Nurse at the middle level of the organisation focusing on teamworking, consistent approaches to care and leadership.

Final reflections

Understanding how care fits into the context of organisations is a first step in being able to lead and manage change as you move through your career as a healthcare professional. As the person with dementia's journey progresses, the organisations we work in need to be responsive and adaptive to deliver person-centred and relationship-centred care.

Further reading

Alzheimer's Association, UK has produced a 'This is me' tool, available at: www.alzheimers.org.uk/site/scripts/download_info.php?downloadID=399 (accessed 02/05/16).

Funded by the National Lottery, the CHOICE project highlights examples of good and not-so-good care and explores each case in context to the organisational culture: The CHOICE (Care Home Organisations Implementing Cultures of Excellence) research report. 025/0064. Available at: www.tsab.org.uk/wp-content/uploads/2015/11/CHOICE_final_report.pdf (accessed 06/03/17).

5

Managing relationship-based approaches to care

Learning objectives

By the end of this chapter, the reader will be able to:

- Examine how to organise the delivery of relationship-based dementia care.
- Explore how leadership and teamworking is influenced by the structure of the organisation as a complex adaptive system.
- Analyse the barriers and enablers at the middle (*meso*) level of the organisation that might impede or promote a dementia-friendly service.
- Construct an individual staff development plan that promotes relationship-based dementia care.

Introduction

Person-centred care is often dependent upon the staff who may be on duty. Alternatively, staff may perceive positive achievements with people with dementia as 'lucky' rather than attributing these achievements to a person-centred strategy. In Chapter 3, we discussed how dementia care was part of a highly regulated industry with formalised and bureaucratic structures and explored how organisations could be viewed as Complex Adaptive Systems (CAS) as a means of promoting relationship-based dementia care. We then examined, in Chapter 4, how these different components would work at the *micro* level of the organisation where we deliver care. We considered the value of biography in planning the care of a person with dementia and how we could encourage the contribution of families to deliver relationship-based dementia care. In this chapter, we will be using the care plan developed in Activity 4.3 to consider how we might work with staff to ensure a consistent approach to relationship-based dementia care.

You don't need to be a manager to use the strategies outlined in this chapter as the ability to lead is needed at all levels of the organisation to ensure we deliver the best care and support for people with dementia and their families. We will explore different aspects of leadership and teamworking that enable teams to articulate how they implement person- or relationship-centred strategies. Taking the lead within teams is often the first step in ensuring care and support is consistent across teams and shifts within an organisation. This activity is generally led at the *meso* level of an organisation and directly influences how care and support is enacted. Managers and Team Leaders are often responsible for delivery of the mission statement of an organisation and in Practice scenario 3.2 we saw that when managers focus on the tasks of care it is unlikely that you will see staff engaging in practice that reflects person-centred care. If the values of the organisation are different to the values of staff who try to influence a more person-centred approach to care, the lack of management responsiveness to staff insights may result in staff feeling demotivated and believing that their input makes no difference (Killett et al., 2016). This may then result in subcultures within an organisation where the values held by different team members act as attractors to bring them together to work in a way that reflects their individual values. This explains why there may be different cultures at unit level within the same organisation.

We will also explore within this chapter leadership and teamworking in more detail through the lens of Complex Adaptive Systems. The key aspects of CAS influenced by management practices at the *meso* level of an organisation are the flow of information across an organisation that facilitates or blocks self-organisation (Anderson et al., 2003). This is not to say that self-organisation will not occur but that it may fail to align with the organisational goals. Anderson and colleagues (2003) found that the following management practices each led to better resident outcomes with a reduction in the prevalence of aggressive behaviour, restraint use, complications of immobility, and fractures:

- Communication openness – being able to share ideas without fear of retribution.
- Participation in decision-making with all perspectives being heard.
- Relationship-oriented leadership is considered necessary in creating interactions between staff and includes giving constructive feedback, helping staff resolve conflict, generating trust and being approachable.

Conversely, Anderson et al. (2003) also found that nursing homes with a higher level of formalisation in working practices that did not promote flexible working resulted in a higher prevalence of complications such as immobility with the over-reliance on rules and enforcement reducing positive relationships between staff (Anderson et al., 2003). These findings suggest that in adopting practices which facilitate self-organisation, care outcomes may improve. However, a limitation of the model of CAS as proposed by Anderson and colleagues is the exclusion of family and resident perspectives as a source of additional information by which staff can make decisions. If we consider care that focuses exclusively on the physical outcomes for residents then it becomes more difficult to identify how families and staff might make valuable contributions. A vital aspect of leadership in dementia care is enabling the perspective of the person with dementia to be heard.

Leadership

Leaders are required at all levels of the organisation to invest in the mission and vision of that organisation. Leaders are not always managers although managers will be expected to demonstrate leadership, particularly when organisational change is required. Leaders influence the culture of the organisation formally when in positions of management and informally when recognised as leaders by the staff within the organisation. Some people may be 'born leaders' but overall, it is generally recognised that leadership requires a set of skills that can be developed. Leadership is currently a feature of many undergraduate nursing curricula with the belief that all nurses need leadership skills to be effective in any organisation in which they practise. When change is needed in an organisation, having effective leaders at all levels of the organisation is necessary. For example, in the US, Marilyn Rantz and colleagues (2013b) found that lack of effective leadership caused teams to fail in some homes, whereas teams with effective leadership, were able to implement change by engaging in regular communication thus enabling all levels of staff to participate in the change process.

In the previous chapters, we have seen that implementing relationship-based approaches to care requires staff to consider innovative and creative solutions in the way they work. To support staff in applying new ways of working, support is needed at the middle (*meso*) level of an organisation since this is where decisions are made in how to manage staffing and resources. *My Home Life* in the UK for example, developed leadership workshops for care home managers to promote quality of care and quality of life in the aged care sector (Owen, 2006). The use of 'Champions' to support staff in implementing person-centred strategies has also been advocated (Brooker and Woolley, 2007; Rosvik et al., 2013). The notion of Dementia Champions is a concept gaining traction in the UK across healthcare environments. Employing dementia specialist practitioners has been used in hospitals as a mechanism to support staff in managing behaviours by role modelling best practice whilst providing education and training for staff in general wards. Equally, in the community, Admiral Nurses in the UK also provide leadership in dementia care.

Activity 5.1 Reflection

In an organisation in which you are practising:

- What is the style of leadership across your organisation?
- Do you or staff colleagues feel able to make suggestions to promote different ways of providing care for people with dementia?
- How is this encouraged/discouraged?
- What leadership practices might improve the sharing of information?

The next question we need to consider is: How might this style of leadership be achieved? There are a multitude of leadership theories – the quantity of which go well beyond the scope of this book. We shall be selective and choose just two leadership strategies to explore: 'Leading by example' and 'Leading from the front' (Brown Wilson, 2009). 'Leading by example' and 'Leading from the front' relate to the different approaches to relationship-based approaches to care discussed in Chapter 3.

Leading by example

Managers being available and visible across the day were typical in homes where 'Leading by example' occurred. Team Leaders were in constant communication with managers, ensuring a free flow of information, creating opportunities to problem solve at the time a solution was required. If staff were concerned about residents they would have opportunistic corridor conversations with the managers and available staff where information was shared, decisions were made and care was altered in a very responsive mode. Staff were then able to self-organise in ways that met the overall aims of the organisation as decisions were discussed and formulated with management involvement. Killett et al. (2016) suggest that leaders in care organisations need to be able to support staff in solving ongoing problems in day-to-day practice which are consistent with the espoused organisational values. Where managers were open to change for the benefit of residents, staff were more likely to report they could implement person-centred practice and subsequently felt more motivated to deliver person-centred care (Killett et al., 2016). Ruth Anderson and colleagues' work on Complex Adaptive Systems also demonstrated that when care staff were able to make decisions based on their knowledge of the resident in a responsive mode then such decisions resulted in better resident outcomes (Anderson et al., 2005b).

Therefore, we might conclude that leadership which supports a flexible approach to work is more likely to promote relationship-centred and person-centred care as staff are enabled to work flexibly, meeting what is important to individual residents whilst ensuring all residents are receiving appropriate care (Anderson et al., 2005a; Brown Wilson, 2009).

Leading from the front

Managers who promoted a more linear structure to the organisation with all communication following a formal route could be described as 'Leading from the front'. In the home where this was clearly demonstrated the focus on risk management outweighed all other approaches and consequently promoted a task-centred approach to care. This was typified by staff being assigned to 'tasks' such as cleaning and cutting all resident's nails at one specific time in the day. This meant that team leaders could keep abreast of the tasks being done and ensure everything was being 'ticked off'. However a tension arose as the manager was encouraging staff to move from a task focus to a person-centred approach. Staff who were following a task-focus approach in line with risk management could not understand why they needed to change this approach since they felt confident that the task focus ensured the safety of those being cared for. Staff would explain to me how they were complying with the written messages received from the manager. This approach contributed to subcultures across the organisation.

Practice scenario 5.1

In one dementia organisation I was involved with there were distinct subcultures within two units that were facilitated by the leadership of the Registered Nurse and Team Leaders on each unit. One subculture was a person-centred approach where leadership was role modelled and staff felt comfortable in approaching the Team Leader for support with residents. Within this subculture, the Registered Nurse was available on the floor for informal interactions, resulting in problem solving. Additionally, the Team Leader believed that the behaviour of the person with dementia was modifiable when the environment and staff actions were modified. Staff learned by example how to approach different residents based on the resident's personality, characteristics and their biographies once this was role modelled by the Team Leader. In this unit, residents appeared settled and engaged with their surroundings, with staff engaging people with dementia in conversation.

In the second unit's subculture, a task focus predominated where the Team Leader prided themselves on being able to deliver good quality physical care where every resident was 'fed, watered and changed' by the end of the shift. On this unit, interactions with the Registered Nurse were limited to information sharing only. Conversely to the first subculture, the Team Leader on this unit believed that the behaviour of the person with dementia was due to their condition and so could not be modified and that people with dementia consciously engaged in these behaviours to be disruptive. This meant there were always unsettled residents and staff engagement was often limited to telling residents to stop annoying others by such behaviour. In this unit, the messages from a bureaucratic approach outweighed other messages of implementing person-centred care due to the values held by the Team Leader. This is not to say that risk management should be a lesser priority nor that all care needs do not require timely completion.

Practice scenario 5.1 demonstrates how subcultures may emerge within an organisation influenced by the values and mental models of those that are responsible for leading practice. The above example may have been due to the limited cognitive diversity in decision-making as each unit was self-supporting with limited opportunities for communication and subsequent sharing of information between units. This scenario suggests it is possible for Registered Nurses to influence approaches to care by being available to discuss issues at the time staff most need support thus promoting a positive experience of care both for people with dementia and staff (Killett et al., 2013). Relationship-oriented leadership has been described as fostering interconnections, enabling problem solving and generating trust within the context of CAS (Anderson et al., 2003). Although the overarching leadership style was 'leading from the front', this home demonstrated how fostering interconnections and enhancing information flow in one unit promoted self-organisation.

Activity 5.2 Reflection

- Return to the care plan you developed in Activity 4.3.
- What leadership strategies are required to achieve this care?
- How might you facilitate the sharing of information contained in this care plan?

To ensure a consistent approach to relationship-based dementia care, there needs to be leadership underpinned by a respect for the person and knowledge of how dementia impacts on such individuals. In the following section, we will explore the 'team effect' of role modelling as a leadership strategy to influence mental models of team members.

Teamwork and consistent care

How teams are formed within an organisation are generally dictated by the management who take into account the overall staffing and the skill mix of staff required to meet the needs of the service users or clients. Organisational culture will influence how groups work within the organisation by the amount of power and control the organisation exerts and subsequently the level of participation in decisions the organisation allows staff to be involved with (Schien, 2010). We have seen that organisations that are Complex Adaptive Systems enable participation in decision-making between staff holding differing levels of expertise by fostering both formal and informal interactions across the organisation (Anderson et al., 2013). In this section, we will explore how the structure and configuration of teams inhibits or promotes participation in decision-making. Participation in this context has been defined as the application of new or existing relationships to share and process information so enabling multiple interpretations to become part of the decision-making process. In Practice scenario 5.1 we saw how staff interpretations concerning the behaviour of the person with dementia contributed to the staff being able to 'make sense' of that behaviour and subsequently make person-centred decisions in practice. When this mental model was based on myths and stereotypes, as outlined in Chapter 1, the decisions made did not support relationship-based dementia care. Although putting staff in teams who work well together would seem to be a good idea, Practice scenario 5.1 demonstrates that when the team is operating with a focus on the task, then person-centred care is unlikely to be enacted. If however, there is a team that is focused on the person and what is known to be important to that person, then the approach may be more person-centred from within that particular team. Additionally, the opportunity to share information may then become a product of the relationships within the team as they operate from similar assumptions about their practice and actively value the information being shared. Considering the features of a CAS, we can conclude that promoting open and responsive communication stimulates participation in decision-making. Involving a greater amount of staff in the decision-making process means that these staff are more likely to develop skills relevant to the decision context and subsequently make more meaningful decisions (Anderson et al., 2013).

Practice scenario 5.2

A new member of staff joined the team and was very much focused on the task as she began working for the organisation. She spoke about the importance of doing a good job and how her motivation was to develop skills to enable her to undertake professional training at a later date. After three months of working with a team that enacted person-centred and relationship-centred care, the same staff member described how she now made decisions based on what was important to the person rather than the tasks that needed to be completed. She also described how when she was unsure, she would be shown how to approach people in different ways, which resulted in better outcomes for the person with dementia. She would then role model person-centred practice for staff who were new to the unit. This team was known to work responsively when the needs of the person with dementia changed with staff having different skills, being prepared to share their knowledge and expertise with the wider team.

Source: based on unpublished data from Brown Wilson (2007).

Practice scenario 5.2 demonstrated openness in communication where team members felt comfortable in asking for help. Being able to recognise that another person might have different skills to bring to the care situation recognised cognitive diversity and allowed adaptive team-working practices, supporting the move towards person-centred care. This approach meant that the experience and skill mix from across the team was being used flexibly to meet the needs of each resident via the spontaneous flow of information between team members (Utley-Smith et al., 2009).

Activity 5.3 Critical Thinking

- Building on Activity 5.2, describe how you would explain the content of the care plan from Activity 4.3 to other members of the team.
- If someone from within the team did not agree with the approach underpinning your care plan, how might you address this?
- How would you ensure all staff were made aware of the care plan so everyone was delivering care consistently?

Teams are generally identified by the management of the organisation and the parameters in which the team works will also be defined at this middle level of the organisation. We saw in the preceding discussion that leadership can happen at the level of managers or within a team of people. Working as part of a team is a necessary aspect of dementia care. Teams will be organised differently depending on the context of care and even the country. For example, in US nursing homes, there are medical and nursing teams working in the same organisation with Registered Nurses being responsible for care planning who may not be involved in direct care (Colon-Emeric et al., 2006). On these occasions, an open flow of information involving all staff in problem solving improved the quality and quantity of information by promoting cognitive diversity, enabling front line staff to feel empowered in making decisions that met the needs of the residents (Colon-Emeric et al., 2006). Similarly in the UK, when front line staff were empowered to take responsibility for resident wellbeing, such staff were able to implement person-centred care (Killett et al., 2016). Certainly when staff in the UK were able to make informal regular connections with registered nursing staff, a more flexible approach to care delivery was seen, producing relationship-based approaches to care (Brown Wilson, 2007). A further example of increasing cognitive diversity and participation in decision making lies in the inclusion of front line care staff in handover meetings where new information can be shared with all members of the team thus improving client care (Colon-Emeric et al., 2006). Killett and colleagues (2016) also suggest that when problem solving is shared between the group and the solutions are person-centred and successful, then it is likely that the person-centred values become more embedded assumptions within the culture of that group.

Another aspect of open communication and participating in decision-making by teams in dementia care concerns family members particularly as the person with dementia's verbal communication changes. Family members can be a valuable source of information bringing a different perspective and so enriching the cognitive diversity of the situation. To work effectively with families, the personal knowledge and biographical knowledge the family member brings may provide key information to support person-centred or relationship-centred care. Valuing this contribution is the first step in working towards shared understandings (Brown Wilson and Davies, 2009) as many families struggle in making the transition to supporting their loved one following admission to a nursing home (Davies and Nolan, 2004) or in an acute care context (Clissett et al., 2013b).

When teams recognised the contribution that families made to the care of the resident, the team also recognised what was important to the family member, such as being kept regularly informed of any changes to the care of the person with dementia, any accidents that might have happened or if the person with dementia's condition changed (Brown Wilson, 2007). Although some families were initially hyper vigilant, once positive relationships developed and they realised that the team was working towards providing personalised care, the families became more trusting (Brown Wilson, 2007). For these relationships to develop, families were seen as making a contribution towards the care which was supporting the team. When teams worked in this way, family members would describe how staff members would respond immediately to issues they raised and reach a resolution, ensuring the family member's contribution was recognised.

For teams to work effectively towards person-centred care, developing role descriptions that articulate participation in decision-making and communication strategies that promote flexible working patterns are needed. If we are asking staff to reframe their focus from the task to the person with dementia, the way role descriptions are framed needs to be reconsidered. If the focus of the role description is purely on the task then asking staff to undertake person-centred or relationship-centred care may be seen as an additional workload. Therefore, developing a role description that describes relationship-based dementia care may be a useful starting point to review how staff approach their role (see Table 5.1).

Ensuring staff are equipped to do their job is the responsibility of the organisation and the staff development plan communicates how staff are valued, which will invariably be influenced by the organisational culture. How staff perceive the

Table 5.1 Example of a relationship-based role description

Biographical approach to care: Respect the lives people have led by listening to the stories people share about their lives. Use photos or belongings to engage in conversations that are meaningful to the person with dementia. Use stories and conversations with the person with dementia and their family to identify significant details in their care and integrate these into everyday routines. Identify meaningful activities that may give the person with dementia pleasure and provide opportunities to engage in these activities. Consider residents who might have similar approaches to life or similar interests and provide opportunities for them to interact and develop relationships. Find out about the person with dementia's social network and what support the community might make in maintaining these relationships.	**Record keeping:** Record important parts of stories that support you in delivering care in a way that matters to the person with dementia and their family. Regular risk assessment of all residents. Document changes in physical, mental or emotional health and subsequent actions taken. Liaise with advance care practitioners about any changes.
Communication: Recognise the person with dementia's experience and validate this experience (if they say 'ouch' ask if it hurts, **not** I am not hurting you). Be honest but sensitive – if a person with dementia asks for someone that is no longer alive, ask if they miss this person and what they remember about them then use this response to lead into another conversation. Do not treat the person as a child and do not use endearments as a blanket approach to everyone; if a person likes to be called by a pet name, then record this and ensure it is appropriately used. Use touch to communicate with people where appropriate to support them emotionally. Ensure you have the person's attention before engaging in loud conversation or care.	**Decision making:** Involve the person with dementia in everyday decisions about their care. Involve the person with dementia in the development of their care plan. Discuss with the person with dementia how they might like to contribute to the life of the community. Work collaboratively with Advanced Care Practitioners to develop an effective care plan.

Leadership and team working:

Support staff to recognise how to deliver care in a way that matters to the person with dementia.

Organise the delivery of care to ensure significant routines for each person are delivered in a way that ensures a positive experience for the person with dementia.

Involve the person with dementia in conversations that might involve changes to routines.

Use medication rounds to assess the physical and emotional state of the person with dementia.

Liaise with direct care workers about changes in behaviour and assess reasons behind this (e.g. pain, potential infections, nutritional state).

Recognise others' and your own skills and support others where help is required – do not always wait to be 'asked' – work with team members to ensure the person with dementia does not become distressed.

Be flexible in approaching the planning of work and discuss with others how the person with dementia responds to care at different points in the day.

Share stories and anecdotes that support others in getting to know the person with dementia and respect the anecdotes shared by others in the team.

Working with families:

Respect the knowledge the family member brings about the person with dementia by integrating this into the care plan.

Speak to the family about the life the person has led, including shared times and memories and use these in conversation with the person with dementia.

Discuss changes in behaviour of the person with dementia with the family respectfully, looking for reasons behind the behaviour.

Support families during visits with conversation 'starters' about what has been going on in the community.

Involve families in the community in ways that are meaningful to them.

As the needs of the person with dementia change, work together with families to develop a care plan that includes their contribution.

Discuss care planning and delivery with the family in a way that values the person with dementia and explain any anomalies in behaviour as a result of the dementia.

Keep families informed of changes and document how this is to be done.

---

relationship between themselves and the organisation may be influenced by the staff development programme. Equally, how staff perceive they are valued may influence how teams work together and subsequently reflect the organisational culture.

Staff development

Enabling staff to work in person-centred ways requires support at the middle level of the organisation as this is where the education and training plans will be developed. In areas that are highly regulated, there will always be mandatory training for all staff and so approaches such as person-centred care may well be considered an additional extra. However, for staff to see this as a recognised way of working, appropriate education and training is vital.

Activity 5.4 Critical Thinking

- Reviewing the example of a relationship-based role description (Table 5.1), identify your training needs to deliver relationship-based dementia care.
- How do you learn best?
- Identify strategies you could employ that would support your personal development in dementia care.
- How would these strategies support your motivation to work with people living with dementia?

We have now reviewed a number of studies that have reflected a variety of ways of enabling staff to employ alternative approaches to dementia care. These strategies are based on facilitation rather than a didactic approach to staff training and include: use of a Dementia Champion given responsibility for finding out biographical information and then sharing this with the team to implement a person-centred approach (Brooker and Woolley, 2007); a mentor employed by the research team to work alongside facility staff (Cooke et al., 2014); a facilitated model of practice development whereby an external facilitator develops strategies with staff, who themselves then implement the strategies (Chenoweth et al., 2009; Brown Wilson et al., 2013). In each of these studies, facilitated and interactive sessions were a common feature. Participants valued interactive, scenario-based and open-discussion formats that enable staff to work with colleagues and hear different perspectives (Cooke et al., 2014). Bringing a number of people together to discuss scenarios promotes cognitive diversity and so enables new information to be developed and shared as part of the training, for future implementation. However, some staff may not see the relevance of facilitated training approaches particularly if they feel they are already implementing person-centred care (Cooke et al., 2014). This can be problematic particularly when working with organisations that may already have clearly espoused philosophies of person-centred care. On these occasions, I have found that a helpful strategy was to facilitate discussions with staff, supporting them to see the importance of everyday activities and routines in their own lives, then inviting staff to consider how people living with dementia might feel about the routines they were experiencing in residential care. Understanding the importance of everyday routines then enabled staff to reconsider how care routines might be developed to take this information for individual residents into account (Brown Wilson et al., 2013).

In many of the multi-level interventions developed, training is a critical component aimed at reframing the staff perspective regarding the person with dementia, encouraging staff to see the value of social interaction and the meaning behind the person with dementia's actions and behaviours (Chenoweth et al., 2009, 2014). Brooker and Woolley (2007), rather than prescribing training, identified that training should also act as a team-building exercise, being fun, practical and based on examples from the clients staff were working with. The use of group work and one-to-one opportunities for discussions including the use of tip sheets was also found to be a helpful strategy for staff (Cooke et al., 2014). Although each of these interventions was well resourced, including experts beyond the home to support delivery of the intervention, not all staff implemented the interventions, particularly where there was a lack of organisational support from managers (Cooke et al., 2014).

Activity 5.5 Reflection

Throughout this chapter, you have considered how you might support other staff in implementing the care plan you developed in Activity 4.3 to ensure there was a consistent approach across teams and shifts. Describe specific activities you would have undertaken as a Registered Nurse to achieve a consistent approach to caring for a person with dementia using the following headings:

- Leadership
- Communication
- Working with families
- Critical decision-making
- Risk management
- Record keeping
- Audit

Conclusion

Leadership can be found at any level of the organisation, and may be invested in management or specialist positions that are given an explicit role for leadership in dementia care. However, leadership can also be enacted informally at the level of direct care. It is especially significant that we seek to identify both formal and informal leaders within an organisation and understand how they support relationship-based approaches to care.

Managers who recognise what makes a good team may use 'attractors' of similar work-based philosophies or personal motivations to make decisions about who works together. However, if these teams do not perceive the relevance of a relationship-based approach to dementia care then practice in such teams may not change. However, to create teams who might not work well together may invariably result in poor care due to dysfunctional teamworking. The process of team building invariably needs decisions to be made in context with the respective organisation. We have seen that staff motivation and the mental models staff hold also influence how teams perform and that using role modelling supported a positive change in staff attitude. This suggests that staff motivation might not necessarily be fixed but could be developed according to the culture of the team in which the person is working. In the following chapter, we will consider the broader or macro level of the organisation and how this impacts on implementing relationship-based dementia care.

Final reflections

The people we work with and those that lead us influence how we implement care for people living with dementia. All involved in healthcare develop mental models based on knowledge, understanding and experience that guide an individual's practice. If these mental models are based on the myths we discussed at the beginning of this book, then this will limit the implementation of relationship-based dementia care. As professionals we also have the capability to provide leadership to others within those teams in which we practise. We can provide leadership by adopting a biographical approach to care planning and then communicating this effectively to others within our teams. This might be to highlight an improvement in the experience of the person living with dementia or through role modelling relationship-based dementia care. The broader culture of the organisation provides important context when we are seeking to promote a consistent approach to dementia care within an organisation.

Further reading

Admiral Nurses in the UK. This website provides an overview of Admiral Nursing, how roles are funded and how to contact Admiral Nurses in the UK. Available at: www.dementiauk.org/how-we-help/admiral-nursing/ (accessed 26/01/17).

Social Care Institute for Excellence Dementia Gateway. This provides a range of resources including training modules on dementia. Available at: www.scie.org.uk/Dementia/ (accessed 26/01/17).

The University of Tasmania provides a free Massive Open Online Course (MOOC) on dementia care. This is a free, easily accessible nine-week online course that builds upon the latest in international research on dementia. Available at: www.utas.edu.au/wicking

6

Creating dementia-friendly services

Learning objectives

By the end of this chapter, the reader will be able to:

- Examine how organisational culture influences the delivery of relationship-based dementia care.
- Analyse the barriers and enablers at the broadest (*macro*) level of the organisation that might impede or promote a dementia-friendly service.
- Identify what changes might be needed at the organisational level to implement a relationship-based care plan.
- Develop an organisational plan for creating a dementia-friendly environment.

Introduction

In Chapter 3, we examined how organisations behaving as Complex Adaptive Systems (CAS) created capacity for staff to self-organise resulting in new and creative ways of working. We related these concepts to the *micro* (Chapter 4) and *meso* (Chapter 5) levels of the organisation, exploring how factors at each level of the organisation influenced everyday dementia care. We analysed how leadership, relationships and diversity of perspectives enabled teams to develop relationship-based dementia care. We explored how mental models influenced teamwork and also developed strategies for ensuring a consistent approach to care was communicated. Communication has been seen at both the *micro* and *meso* levels of an organisation as both a facilitator and a barrier to person-centred and relationship-centred care. Informal, open and responsive communication patterns involving multiple perspectives enabled problem solving, which contributed to self-organisation. Self-organisation enabled teams to work together to meet the needs of the person with dementia, their families and staff, and was influenced by the culture and leadership of the team. Culture can be described as 'the way things are done around here' and we have seen how this is communicated in direct care, in teams and through leadership. We now turn our attention to the *macro* level of an organisation as 'setting the scene' for the culture of an organisation. At the macro level of the organisation, policies, processes and financial decisions all influence the ability staff have to deliver person-centred or relationship-centred care for the person with dementia. This chapter considers how the macro level of an organisation has the potential to become a facilitator of improved dementia care contributing towards a dementia-friendly service. By examining the broader organisational context in which we work, we are able to identify the key facilitators and barriers that may be impeding the implementation of relationship-based dementia care. The purpose of this chapter is to reframe our perspective of the organisation as a separate entity to one where the *macro* level of the organisation is part of the solution as we endeavour to improve the care and support for people living with dementia and their families. As well as policies and processes, we will also explore the physical environment as changes at this level will have a direct impact on the care delivery and wellbeing of the person with dementia.

Organisational culture

Organisational culture is a contested domain underpinned by diverse assumptions and evidence and may be considered at both a structural and process level (Scott et al., 2003). As we endeavour to implement relationship-based dementia care, we will adopt a definition of organisational culture where the key focus is on relationships. Edgar Schein is considered an expert in this field and has worked with many organisations to implement culture change. He considers organisational culture as the patterns of beliefs, assumptions and behaviours reflecting a commonality between people in an organisation that are constantly re-enacted and created by interactions with others, shaped by an individual's behaviour (Schein, 2010). This definition suggests that culture is a product of interaction through the process of working with others as part of an organisation. These beliefs and assumptions may be influenced by the philosophy and values of an organisation, with interactions being influenced by the physical infrastructure, routine behaviours, language and rituals (Schein, 2010). The physical layout, the rituals and generally what is visible is defined as the surface level of culture with a deeper level of embedded assumptions underneath that people are generally not aware of but will influence their behaviour and so continue to shape the organisational culture (see Figure 6.1).

Organisational culture is usually formally reflected in artefacts such as the mission statement, espoused values, policies and procedures. Alongside this there is also an informal culture generally comprised of symbols, ceremonies, rites and stories. Indeed, there are models of residential aged care that start with making changes to the physical environment such as introducing plants, animals or creating themed corridors that promote sensory stimulation. Smaller group living homes are also being developed and evaluated (see Table 6.1). Many of these models offer support and endorsement for a subscription fee. However, in a recent systematic review of endorsement models, there were limited independent evaluations, with limited evidence of improved outcomes for residents and families (Petriwskyj et al., 2016b).

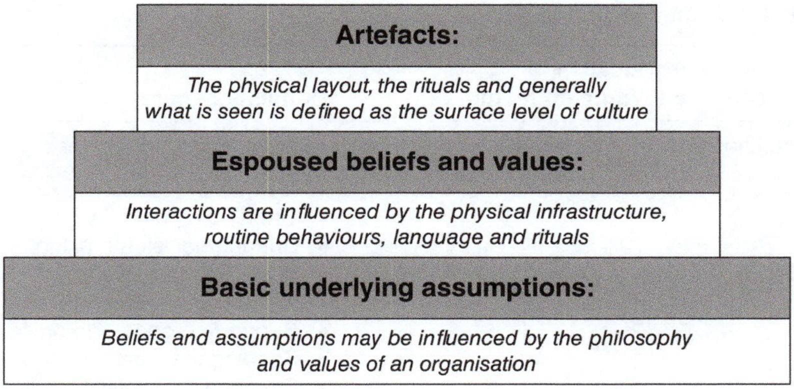

Artefacts:
The physical layout, the rituals and generally what is seen is defined as the surface level of culture
Espoused beliefs and values:
Interactions are influenced by the physical infrastructure, routine behaviours, language and rituals
Basic underlying assumptions:
Beliefs and assumptions may be influenced by the philosophy and values of an organisation

Figure 6.1 Following Schein (2010), the three levels of culture

Whilst the physical environment is easily identifiable, how physical artefacts transfer into the culture of the organisation is more problematic. For example, when staff were asked about changes in some of the models, they were unable to articulate the way these changes had altered their approach to care (Bellot, 2007). A greater understanding of the drivers at the macro level can support us in understanding how the culture of an organisation can be translated into everyday

Table 6.1 Overview of different cultural models of residential dementia care
Based on Petriwskyj et al., 2016a

Model of care	Physical environment features	Domains of care
Eden (US)	Edenisation of the home includes introduction of pets, plants and children.	• Identity • Growth • Autonomy • Security • Connectedness • Meaning • Joy
Greenhouse (US)	The core concept of a green-house is to create smaller living environments for elders that revolve around a centralised 'hearth' with bedrooms coming off the central dining and lounge room areas.	1. Resident direction 2. Home environment 3. Staff empowerment 4. Collaborative decision making

(Continued)

Table 6.1 (Continued)

Model of care	Physical environment features	Domains of care
My Home Life		Eight best practice themes • Maintaining identity • Creating community • Sharing decision making • Managing transitions • Improving health and healthcare • Supporting good end of life • Keeping workforce fit for purpose • Promoting a positive culture
Dementia Care Matters (UK)	Dementia design principles are utilised in partnership with staff, residents and families to improve quality of life of the person with dementia and experience of staff and families.	Household model of care where the person with dementia's reality is accepted and staff are trained in emotional intelligence and to increase positive moments. Leadership and coaching encourage change by supporting staff.
PEARL (UK)	Themed corridors are created that provide opportunities for meaningful activity as the person with dementia walks around the environment alongside creative activities being developed.	Supporting the transition to a care home and getting to know the person through life story work. Promoting positive person work as the foundation of person-centred care, promoting nutrition, engaging in meaningful activity and ensuring good end of life care.

care for people with dementia and their families. More businesses are adopting a consumer model of care and understanding what this language means can support healthcare professionals in developing care practice in line with organisational goals.

Activity 6.1 Reflection

In an organisation in which you practise:

1 Explore the formal culture:

- Find a mission statement – how does this reflect the values you are trying to achieve when caring for people with dementia in this organisation?
- What does the physical layout communicate towards people with dementia?
- How do the rituals (e.g. personal care, meal times) value the person with dementia?

2 Explore the informal culture:

- How do people talk about the person with dementia?
- How is this different or similar to the mission statement of the organisation?
- Do the stories people tell about activities within the organisation reflect the mission statement?
- Does the physical layout facilitate a relationship-based approach to care?

The physical environment – cultural artefacts

The environments we live in become of greater importance as people age. For many years, ageing in place has been seen as important for older people. This has meant that homes are now being designed with adaptations for long term disability thus supporting people with diminishing capabilities to age in place. The provision of care options has also seen the development of retirement villages offering a range of care options that people may access as they age. However, limited supported living options exist for the person with dementia who wishes to live in the community rather than a residential facility. This makes the development of dementia-friendly environments more pressing.

Artefacts such as the physical environment can be used to communicate the culture of a service. People being able to bring in important possessions from their own home, having plants and a pet alongside opportunities to have meals with visiting family members represent the creation of a home-like environment. In this way, people with dementia, families and staff are drawn into the organisation. For example, in residential environments, creating physical spaces where people can find a quiet space for private time or visits with friends and family clearly demonstrates to everyone that the culture is one that is trying to create a home-like environment. However, for a person living with dementia, the purpose of incorporating dementia-friendly design into the physical environment is to minimise the impairments that come with the condition of dementia and so not further disable the person. For example, being unable to find your way or orientate yourself to your surroundings impacts on how you feel about yourself. This can have a detrimental effect on a person with dementia's wellbeing since being unable to find their way around implies a lack of mastery over something normally very simple. Dependency upon others may also be created as help is required to navigate the physical environment and being unable to find their way around would not give a person a sense that they belong in that environment. This is an area that will be governed by finance at the *macro* level of an organisation. The level of investment suggests the importance of people with dementia within an organisation, but to create a more accommodating environment may not always need major changes. It may be as simple as changing the lighting and/or décor to aid wayfinding of the person with dementia.

In Australia, Davis and colleagues (2009) suggest that a positive physical environment enables the person with dementia to engage with others in both meaningful relationships and meaningful activities and so remain active participants in residential environments. This can be achieved by the design of a bedroom that enables a person to enjoy private time with family and friends or small kitchen areas that enable the person with dementia to continue to participate in meaningful activity around meal times. Davis et al. (2009) suggest that long-term care provides seven living experiences based on the physical design but also influenced by the social interactions that occur: the presentation of self-experience, eating experience, personal enjoyment experience, bedroom experience, family and community connections experience, end-of-life experience and the staff experience. An analysis of data from over 200 people with dementia across 35 care homes in Sydney demonstrated a statistically significant correlation between quality of life (QoL) and the physical environment (Fleming et al., 2016). The most important features of the environment for QoL included a path that took the person past interesting activities, access to private areas, and opportunities to engage in social interaction along with everyday activities of daily living (Fleming et al., 2016).

Practice scenario 6.1

A medium-sized not-for-profit care organisation in the UK developed a dementia-friendly service by involving myself as an academic with experience in dementia care, architects, a care manager and a business manager. Incorporating these perspectives into the design process means that the design would reflect the dementia care model of delivery being developed. Evidence-based design principles for people living with dementia were accessed from the University of Stirling. This ensured the built environment was functional in supporting the needs of people living with dementia. In this process, difficult decisions were made as to what was the most important aspect in facilitating the best experience for the person with dementia, given other (including financial) constraints. A small kitchen on each floor was included that enabled the person with dementia to be involved in the serving of food at meal times or where they could cook themselves or offer hospitality to their visitors. Open plan spaces were developed enabling furniture to be arranged according to the function of the space – i.e. a quiet corner, a place for watching television, a place for sitting with others. This design feature prevented the structure of the room lending itself to chairs being placed along walls, often identified as a poor design feature in residential environments. Other design features included the use of contrasting colours between walls and doors to identify or obscure doorways; the use of plain carpet to avoid illusions of steps or water on the floor; clear and appropriate signage to facilitate the person with dementia's engagement with their environment.

Outdoor spaces and connecting to nature is integral to people with dementia (Gilliard and Marshall, 2012). In residential environments, outdoor spaces are also pivotal for people with dementia and there is a growing body of knowledge that demonstrates the benefits for the person with dementia in being able to remain actively engaged with outdoor spaces. There is also evidence of social, psychological and health benefits for people with dementia from spending time outdoors, the healing power of nature, activities in the garden, animals, multisensory exercise, and the use of nature to explore memories. Work undertaken by Garuth Chalfont (2006) demonstrated evident benefits in the interaction, initiation, concentration and activity completion for the person with dementia. Dementia Adventure is an example of a UK company specialising in supporting people with dementia and their caregivers to undertake outdoor activities from visiting historic houses and their gardens to sailing and hiking holidays. Maintaining a connection to the outdoors is a core part of spirituality – in my previous book, we considered that spirituality was more than religiosity and was about realising there was something greater than you. Understanding how a person with dementia interacts with the outdoor environment is an important part of ensuring meaningful activity as nature-based activities improve psychological and physical wellbeing (Chalfont, 2006).

Providing external spaces to interact with nature or continue gardening activities enables continuity with a previous life. Gardening as part of the home environment may mean different things to different people. However, domestic spaces such as the garden affect self-determination and promote a sense of continuity and choice. However, people with dementia may need support to access outdoor spaces as the following practice scenario suggests.

Practice scenario 6.2

Edward was an avid gardener and had recently been admitted to a dementia-friendly ward where a garden had been created. Staff observed that Edward enjoyed sitting in the garden but they rarely had any staff to supervise him in case he fell. Adopting a multidisciplinary approach, a plan was constructed for a physiotherapist to assess Edward's walking in the garden and provide exercises to reduce the risk of falls, and an Occupational Therapist to work with Edward to reach mastery of horticultural activities he would enjoy. Following this plan, staff working in the ward could facilitate this activity once Edward was able to undertake it independently.

Risk is part of everyday life and people with dementia should be enabled to engage in activities even where there is risk. This might require input from a multidisciplinary team such as in the case of Edward. A key feature in the practice scenario above was changing the perception of staff to recognise the value of meaningful activity within the daily routine. This has the potential for staff to then facilitate more opportunities for people with dementia to enjoy outdoor spaces and activity.

Dementia-friendly design is also needed in hospitals as this environment can be a particularly disorienting experience for people living with dementia and their caregivers. A number of studies have suggested that people with dementia admitted to hospitals have poorer outcomes than those without dementia and so the Department of Health in the UK commissioned the Kings Fund to undertake projects to enhance the environment of care to improve the patient experience. This resulted in over 250 projects across a range of health and social care organisations, with an additional 25 projects in acute hospitals and Mental Health Trusts being completed in 2010 (Waller et al., 2013).

Practice scenario 6.3

Enhancing the Healing Environment case study

The aim of the project was to create a more therapeutic environment to increase patients' wellbeing by improvements to the entrance, corridors and main social space in this dementia assessment unit.

The entrance has been redesigned to provide a friendly, spacious, welcoming first impression with an open reception desk and comfortable seating for visitors. Patients and carers were involved in choosing the poems and words that decorated the walls.

Internally, patients' orientation was improved with the use of colour and numbers on each of the bedroom doors together with a series of commissioned artworks in the corridors.

The main day and dining space has been subdivided so that seating was arranged in small clusters. As part of the project the team reviewed how space was being used and a number of other improvements to the ward area were made including the creation of a carers' room and kitchen space for occupational therapy activities.

Source: www.kingsfund.org.uk/projects/enhancing-healing-environment/completed-projects/cumbria-partnership-nhs-foundation-trust (accessed 27/01/17).

Small-scale evaluations of the Enhancing the Healing Environments projects indicate that there has been progress in developing more dementia-friendly environments including the securing of finance to improve the physical environment of care such as improving signage, flooring, lighting and colour schemes as part of maintenance programmes and making small-scale improvements such as purchasing coloured crockery.

Activity 6.2 Reflection

In the organisation in which you practise what are some of the difficulties a person with dementia might have in finding their way to the following areas?

- Toilet
- Bedroom
- Dining room
- Outdoor area

What changes could be made to improve this experience?

Another set of artefacts that influence the culture of an organisation are documents such as a vision or mission statement that then influences policies developed across the organisation. In this context, the concept of 'attractors' as a mechanism for agents (people with dementia, families and staff) within the organisation to be drawn to each other with a common goal is one that can be used meaningfully at the macro level. For example, a policy that clearly articulates what person-centred dementia care means both at a strategic level as well as at a practical level can be used by managers and staff as a focal point to guide everyday decisions about practice. Killett et al. (2016) found that when there were consistent organisational policies and procedures in place, person-centred activity and engagement became integral to care work.

Activity 6.3 Critical thinking

- Access a policy in your organisation and compare it to the policy below.
- What changes need to be made to reflect person-centred principles?

Example of a policy using the language of person-centred care

Practice guidance for implementation of person-centred care

- This practice guidance is based on guidelines for best practice [1] and practice-based research [2].
- A full assessment of the needs of the person should be undertaken with reference to their past life with a discussion identifying meaningful activities and significant routines they have maintained in their lives.
- A profile of community and/or activity links should be generated to be able to discuss appropriate meaningful activities for the person's activities.
- The person with dementia and significant others should be included in the decision-making process with best interest meetings conducted as appropriate to ensure the person with dementia is able to maintain links with community and their other interests as part of their weekly routines.
- Attention to detail: significant details that may have an adverse impact on the person with dementia if they are not maintained should be prioritised. Use care routines to initiate conversation about the person's life and/or their interests as this will enable them to enter into meaningful conversation with you and share information you may not know about them [2].
- Changes in behaviour should be considered in respect to the daily care routines or significant events in a person's life and how this might be influencing these changes.
- Changes in behaviour should also be considered in respect to changes in a person's eating, drinking, mobility, continence, or emotional state suggesting a change in physical health such as pain or infection (such as urinary tract infection or chest infection for example). If a physical condition is suspected, immediate referral is required to the nominated healthcare professional.
- Anticipating needs: knowing a person's daily routine and what is important to them in their day will support an understanding of what 'might come next' and what might

(Continued)

(Continued)

be the likely outcome if this usual routine is not maintained. Using this information to organise care for a number of people you may have responsibility for will help to avoid difficulties when a person with dementia (or their family member) might not understand why a change to their routine is required [2].

Record keeping

- Storytelling is an appropriate method of communication by a person with dementia and their families. Staff are responsible for identifying significant details in the story being told as it relates to care and activity routines. This should be recorded in the person's care records and the care plan amended as appropriate [2].
- All daily care records need to communicate the impact of activities or changes of interest within the activity so that patterns might be identified that may signal a change to the activity programme is required.
- Record keeping should include a person's social and emotional health including how they feel, how they are responding in situations and issues relating to the wellbeing of the person.

References

[1] National Collaborating Centre for Mental Health (2007) *Dementia*. A NICE–SCIE guideline on supporting people with dementia and their carers in health and social care. National Clinical Practice Guideline Number 42. The British Psychological Society and Gaskell.

[2] Brown Wilson, C. and Davies, S. (2009) Using relationships in care homes to develop relationship-centred care – the contribution of staff. *Journal of Clinical Nursing*, 18, 1746–1755.

Involving all stakeholder voices

Focusing on the macro level of an organisation, there are key agents in the senior management teams at executive level and on management boards in larger organisations that will have overarching responsibility for the company. It is generally at this level that changes to vision and resourcing are made. However, to maintain the focus of decisions in a small group of people at this point would be to inhibit change and potentially prevent meaningful change at the *meso* and *micro* levels of the organisation. Cognitive Diversity has been a common theme in Complex Adaptive Systems, discussed in previous chapters. Involving multiple perspectives promotes the emergence of new thinking. This means staff at all levels of the organisation should be involved in the decisions but this should also extend to include the person with dementia and their families. As part of the regulatory requirements in the UK, care organisations need to involve residents and their families in decisions that affect them. These aspects of decision-making are generally considered to remain in the domain of direct care; however, bringing these same stakeholders' perspectives to be included at the macro level of organisational decision-making is one way to increase cognitive diversity and ensure all perspectives are considered. Difficulties commonly experienced in dementia such as communication and memory loss may be used as an excuse for not involving people living with dementia at the macro level of the organisation. However, there are people living with early or middle stages of dementia in the community that could support the work of Boards and CEO's on a regular basis. The configuration of the Board is vital in ensuring a range of perspectives as both business and clinical perspectives need to be represented at the top decision-making table. Many people living with dementia in a residential environment may struggle with written and verbal communication and may not be able to complete surveys or participate in focus groups but are still able to communicate what works for them. Finding innovative ways of including the views of a person with dementia on a routine basis rather than as a one-off event is needed if all perspectives are going to be included in the decision-making process.

Practice scenario 6.4

One organisation I worked with firmly believed in supporting staff and involving the people they cared for in decision-making. This was transferred into involving service users in round table discussions at key points in the year, which was then fed into the operational team meetings of senior managers. This information was then communicated to the Executive Board and used in decision-making. Staff surveys were also distributed annually and the executive team would visit all service areas over the course of the year to speak directly with staff delivering services. This company also operated a virtual 'suggestion box' with prizes given to staff for good ideas. An awards ceremony occurred every year where good practice in line with the mission and vision of the organisation was rewarded for both individuals and teams.

Developing a dementia-friendly community

We have seen in this chapter that environments for people with dementia requiring care and support are being re-conceptualised with a focus on the experience from the perspective of the person living with dementia (Davis et al., 2009). A dementia-friendly community is one in which people with dementia feel they can contribute and participate in activities that are meaningful to them. Not every organisation will create a community in the same way. For some it will be about supporting people with dementia to access the wider community environment and for others it will be about promoting community within a home-like residential environment. The purpose of a dementia-friendly environment is to minimise the impairments that come with the condition of dementia and so not disable the person. This will then support the person living with dementia in maintaining their independence and quality of life rather than being a passive recipient of care (Davis et al., 2009).

Practice scenario 6.5

Dementia villages have been designed in the Netherlands enabling the person with dementia to remain engaged and active within their chosen lifestyle in a community. The villages feature small group homes with access to a safe community environment including a supermarket, a theatre and restaurants. This enables the person with dementia to live a life of their choosing, enabled rather than disabled by the environment. This suggests it is helpful to see the physical environment as a means of enablement rather than an end point. In effect, the physical environment is the location in which lives are lived, relationships are formed and meaningful activities undertaken.

Source: http://hogeweyk.dementiavillage.com/en/kenniscentrum/ (accessed 27/01/17).

Mitchell and colleagues (2004) worked with 20 older people with dementia and 25 without dementia to determine the characteristics of the built environment that supported or discouraged people with dementia from engaging with their community environment. This study found that even in familiar environments, areas such as street crossings caused people with dementia to lose their way by providing too much information resulting in disorientation. Many people with dementia in this study chose routes that were varied, with smaller roads that enabled them to maintain concentration; they tended to avoid uniform areas or long wide straight roads as these became difficult to navigate due to a lack of distinguishing environmental landmarks. In interviews with people with dementia, a preference was expressed for simple signs on a light background to aid wayfinding. Too many signs or signs with too much information were not seen as helpful.

A report by the Alzheimer's Society in 2013 clearly identifies the importance of hearing the voices of people living with dementia and their caregivers in the design of dementia-friendly communities. Worryingly, only 35% of people with dementia surveyed said they left their house once a week with 65% not feeling able to try new things due to a lack of confidence, worry and fear; 66% of these people also stated they did not feel able to make a contribution to the community although they believed they could contribute in a meaningful way. There are 10 key areas that dementia-friendly communities should be working towards (see Table 6.2).

Table 6.2 Dementia-friendly communities

Dementia-friendly communities	
Involvement of people with dementia	Shape communities around the needs and aspirations of people living with dementia alongside the views of their carers.
Challenge stigma and build understanding	Work to break down the stigma of dementia, including in seldom heard communities, and increase awareness and understanding of dementia.
Accessible community activities	Offer organised activities that are specific and appropriate to the needs of people with dementia. Also ensure that existing leisure services and entertainment activities are more inclusive of people with dementia.
Acknowledge potential	Ensure that people with dementia themselves acknowledge the positive contribution they can make to their communities. Build on the goodwill in the general public to make communities dementia friendly.
Ensure an early diagnosis	Ensure access to early diagnosis and post-diagnostic support. Have health and social care services that are integrated and delivering person-centred care for people with dementia in all settings.
Practical support to enable engagement in community life	Deliver a befriending service that includes practical support to ensure people with dementia can engage in community life as well as offering emotional support.
Community-based solutions	Support people with dementia in whatever care setting they live, from maintaining independence in their own home to inclusive, high-quality care homes.
Consistent and reliable travel options	Community-based solutions to housing can prevent people from unnecessarily accessing healthcare and support people to live longer in their own homes.
Easy-to-navigate environments	Ensure that the physical environment is accessible and easy to navigate for people with dementia.
Respectful and responsive businesses and services	Promote awareness of dementia in all shops, businesses and services so all staff demonstrate understanding and know how to recognise symptoms.
	Encourage organisations to establish strategies that help people with dementia utilise their business.

Source: www.actonalz.org/sites/default/files/documents/Dementia_friendly_communities_full_report.pdf pp. 41–42 (accessed 25/01/17).

Activity 6.4 Action

Develop an organisational plan for creating a sense of community within a dementia-friendly environment utilising the following:

- Mission statement
- Values and attitudes
- Staff motivation
- Physical environment

Conclusion

Organisations are constantly evolving and need to keep up with changes both externally and internally. Designing dementia-friendly environments taking into account the perspective of people living with dementia is being recognised as best practice in providing person-centred care. This might be in new builds or by improving signage and wayfinding opportunities in existing buildings. Mission statements and policy documents are important artefacts that shape the culture of an organisation. The values and language of person-centred care need to be reflected at the macro level of the organisation.

Final reflections

Across the last three chapters we have considered how to implement relationship-based approaches to care within our everyday care at the micro level of the organisation, then how working as part of a team with the attendant leadership enables a flexible and responsive pattern of care, facilitating relationship-based approaches to care at the meso level of the organisation. In this chapter we have considered the broader or macro context in organisations focusing on the influence policies and the physical environment have on our ability to implement relationship-based approaches to care. In the following chapters, we will return to the micro level as we focus on the person with dementia and their families.

Further reading

Culture change models

These websites provide additional details and resources related to the respective philosophies identified in Table 6.1:

www.edenalt.org (accessed 27/01/17).

myhomelife.org.uk (accessed 27/01/17).

www.dementiacarematters.com/our_dementia_care_philosophy.html (accessed 27/01/17).

Sustain

Sustain is an alliance that advocates food and agriculture policies and practices that enhance the health and welfare of people and animals, improve the working and living environment, enrich society and culture and promote equity. Sustain represents around 100 national public interest organisations working at international, national, regional and local level. Resources are provided for engaging people with dementia in gardening and horticulture:

www.sustainweb.org/(accessed 27/01/17).

www.sustainweb.org/resources/files/reports/Dementia_Factsheet.pdf (accessed 27/01/17).

Dementia-friendly environments

The Dementia Services Development Centre at the University of Stirling has developed evidence-based design ideas to create dementia-friendly environments. This includes the principles and how to implement them as well as audit toolkits and a consultancy service:

http://dementia.stir.ac.uk/design (accessed 27/01/17).

http://dementia.stir.ac.uk/design/virtual-environments/virtual-hospital (accessed 27/01/17).

http://dementia.stir.ac.uk/design/virtual-environments/virtual-care-home (accessed 27/01/17).

Australian example of seven dementia design principles

The State of Victoria in Australia funded a dementia-friendly project that resulted in the development of seven key indicators for a dementia-friendly environment. Resources have subsequently been developed to support aged care organisations to improve the lived experience in these areas. For more details, see: https://www2.health.vic.gov.au/ageing-and-aged-care/dementia-friendly-environments (accessed 27/01/17).

Chalfont design

Dr Garuth Chalfont is widely recognised as an expert in supporting people with dementia in accessing outdoor spaces and supporting staff in being able to integrate outdoor spaces into their care. There are a range of resources for the development of therapeutic gardens: www.chalfontdesign.com/

The Kings Fund

Enhancing the Healing environment, available at: www.kingsfund.org.uk/projects/enhancing-healing-environment/ehe-design-dementia (accessed 25/01/17).

Developing supportive design for people with dementia, available at: www.kingsfund.org.uk/projects/enhancing-healing-environment (accessed 25/01/17).

7

Developing community through dementia-friendly environments

> **Learning objectives**
>
> By the end of this chapter, the reader will be able to:
>
> - Examine the key principles of a positive personal and social environment for people living with dementia.
> - Explore how the environment (personal, social and physical) may influence the behaviour of a person with dementia.
> - Develop a relationship-centred care plan for a person who may be experiencing Behavioural and Psychological Symptoms of Dementia (BPSD).
> - Identify a relevant educational strategy for your area of practice that will support staff in adopting a relationship-based approach to care.

Introduction

We have used the lens of Complex Adaptive Systems to examine how relationship-based dementia care has the potential to be delivered at all levels of the organisation. In the previous chapter, we explored how the culture of an organisation was established and the role the physical environment played in enabling people with dementia. Being unable to find your way or orientate yourself to your surroundings can have a detrimental effect on an individuals' wellbeing. For example, a lack of mastery of something this fundamental in everyday life impacts on a person's sense of belonging in that environment. For the person with dementia, this can create dependency as help is required to navigate the physical environment. In the previous chapter we reviewed what a dementia-friendly environment would look like in a range of organisations. However, environment is not just about the physical space but also about the relationships we develop and the people we interact with. In earlier chapters, we noted how the culture of an organisation sets the scene for teamwork and how care is delivered demonstrating the integral nature of relationships in the implementation of person-centred or relationship-centred care.

In this chapter we will consider the personal and social environment from the perspective of the person with dementia. A person's life experience or biography creates an internal environment that may influence how the person with dementia behaves in different social situations. Thus understanding the biography of a person with dementia supports us in understanding their personal environment. For example, knowing how a person used to react to situations that made them feel uncomfortable before they had dementia may provide insight into why a person reacts as they do to a current situation. As people with dementia lose ability to express themselves in the usual way, they may struggle to communicate how they are feeling and so respond with behaviour that staff and families find challenging. Such behaviour could be a result of an emotional response triggered by an interaction between the personal, social and/or physical environment in which the person finds himself/herself. However, if this behaviour is seen as communication, there is the potential for staff to reinterpret the behaviour. Adapting this knowledge to support the person with dementia in everyday practice could be in anticipating situations we know the person might find uncomfortable and thus considering ways of minimising the adverse impact of the situation by responding flexibly to the needs of the person and others within the environment. In this context, the behaviour is no longer interpreted as challenging by the staff but encourages them to consider alternative ways of promoting wellbeing for the person with dementia.

Relationships between people with dementia, their families and staff all contribute towards the social environment of an organisation. The social environment is not static but interlinked and in a constant state of movement. The social environment is influenced by the team that is on duty, how people with dementia are responding to the situation, levels of stress experienced by staff, family visits and how staff perceive interactions with families. Developing a critical mass of staff in and across teams that understand the behaviours being demonstrated and who can respond positively promotes shared understandings that then contributes to a sense of community. Creating a sense of community requires consistent leadership at all levels of the organisation: *macro*, *meso* and *micro*. Leadership is a critical role for Team Leaders as they support staff in responding flexibly to changing situations thus promoting the wellbeing of the person with dementia. Understanding how the personal, social and physical environment may affect the person with dementia is central to anticipating needs irrespective of the location. To facilitate the application to practice of this knowledge, this chapter presents a range of evidence-based resources that can be used to support all staff in promoting a sense of community.

Creating a positive personal and social environment

In Chapter 6, we considered person-centred philosophies at the broader organisational level but if staff are not supported to implement these, then person-centred care might not always be enacted in practice (Moyle et al., 2013b). In Chapter 5, we explored the role of teams and the importance of team leadership to facilitate a relationship-based approach to care. Leadership through role modelling relationship-based approaches to care promoted a critical mass of staff with shared values resulting in a team that delivered consistent care (Brown Wilson, 2009). These relationship-based approaches to dementia care begin with the biography of the person. Listening to and integrating these stories into everyday care routines is the first step in developing personal and responsive relationships (Brown Wilson et al., 2009). Positive relationships enable staff to value the stories being shared and thus adopt a biographical approach to care. The next step in supporting people living with dementia is to understand how their biography contributes to their behaviour. We often believe we understand the life history of a person by knowing their marital or partnership status, their employment history, where they have lived and their family connections. However, in a small practice development project I was involved with, it was increasingly evident that keeping knowledge at this level was insufficient to implement person-centred care. Activity 7.1 is designed to support you in understanding what these aspects of a person's biography mean for the person with dementia.

Activity 7.1 Reflection

1. Draw a line and plot your life history – include events that have significance to you and events that have shaped who you are today.
2. How have these events shaped the way you live:
   - i What makes you feel comfortable in your home?
   - ii What gives you a sense of being linked to your past?
   - iii What connects you to family and friends?
3. How have these events shaped the way you react to the following situations:
   - iv If you get frustrated with something – how do you react and why?
   - v If you feel uncomfortable with a situation – how do you react and why?
   - vi If you feel happy – how do you react and why?

- Consider a person with dementia you are supporting or have supported; undertake the same activity with them.
- How has this developed your understanding of this person?

From Activity 7.1, we can see how events shape who we are and how we might respond to certain situations. Clare Surr (2006) identified how people with dementia use metaphors to explain their understanding of the current situation and these stories maintain a connection to the person's sense of self. Certainly in places I have worked, these stories are often discounted as a person being confused in time or place. However Surr (2006) contends that stories recounted by the person with dementia are a mechanism of communication and may be communicating anxiety or fears, which becomes particularly important when the person with dementia's executive function is no longer intact. This means that the person may not have the same ability to modify or moderate their behaviour as they once did. However, this doesn't mean that behaviours are not without significance.

A key feature of supporting people with dementia are the behavioural and psychological symptoms that come with the condition. Behaviours, for example, may mean a person with dementia is in pain, or they are anxious, depressed or distressed. There is no one recipe for what different behaviours mean, however all behaviours need to be seen within the context of the person's biography and the place in which they live. A change in behaviour may initially be recognised as the person not being their 'usual self'. Whilst this is a valid observation, being able to articulate what this means is the next step if the appropriate care is to be received.

Behavioural and psychological symptoms

Many people with dementia experience disturbed perception resulting in behavioural and psychological symptoms of dementia (BPSD) which include agitation, anxiety, mood disorders, aberrant motor behaviour, delusions, hallucinations, disinhibition and sleep or appetite changes (Cerejeira et al., 2012) (see Table 7.1). A person with dementia may exhibit a range of behaviours simultaneously, creating difficulty in the assessment and subsequent treatment of BPSD. Not treating BPSD can significantly reduce quality of life for both the person with dementia and their caregivers. Distinguishing between different symptoms can be challenging when dementia is a comorbid condition – for example, depression and apathy may be misinterpreted as being represented by the same behaviour (Cerejeira et al., 2012). Large cohort studies of BPSD in people with dementia demonstrate that if people have symptoms at one point in time, they are also likely to have symptoms later in the disease process. The most common symptoms are mood disorders (depression and apathy): with depression tending to improve and apathy worsening as the dementia advances (Aalten et al., 2005a). Although people with dementia are less able to articulate how they feel, their behaviours can continue to be observed. In a prospective longitudinal cohort study by Aalten and colleagues (2005b) the most consistent behaviour over the course of dementia was aberrant motor behaviour which worsened over time in patients with moderate dementia.

Table 7.1 Behavioural and psychological symptoms based on Cerejeira et al. (2012)

Syndrome (Aalten et al., 2003)	Symptoms	Examples of behaviour
Mood/apathy	Depression	Feelings of sadness or hopelessness; additional activity or reduced activity
	Anxiety	Expressions that demonstrate the person is worried, repetitive questioning expressing concerns
	Heightened emotional states	Constant movement or no movement initiated
Psychosis	Delusions	False belief of someone stealing
	Disturbed perceptions	Hallucinations
Hyperactive behaviour	Agitation	Physically non-aggressive Verbally non-aggressive Physically aggressive Verbally aggressive
	Repetitive purposeless behaviour	Asking the same question, or shadowing the caregiver
	Socially inappropriate behaviours	Disinhibition Wandering away from the home
Sleep disturbance	Insomnia, hypersomnia, disordered REM sleep	Sleeping in the day and being awake at night
Appetite disturbance	Change in taste Loss of appetite	Refusing to eat foods once enjoyed

Source: based on Cerejeira et al. (2012).

A person with dementia may be experiencing more than one symptom at the same time, with some conditions overlapping. For example, repetitive wandering behaviours my impact on a person's ability to sit and complete a meal, which in turn may give rise to weight loss. Alternatively, apathy and depression may be misinterpreted as they appear similar in behaviour.

Careful consideration should always be applied when we think about behaviour in relation to the person with dementia and there are two widely used models that can be used to underpin our practice: Need-Driven Dementia-Compromised Behaviour Model (NDB) and Progressively Lowered Stress Threshold Model.

Need-Driven Dementia-Compromised Behaviour Model (NDB) was developed by Algase and colleagues in 1996 and starts from the premise that the behaviour of a person with dementia is driven by a need or a goal that is relevant to that person with dementia. This premise removes the label often associated with difficult behaviours that staff consider challenging and also prevents the stigma of labelling someone as 'aggressive'. The underlying problem with these types of labels is that staff begin to associate these behaviours with a particular person and then consider all behaviours as problematic rather than looking behind the behaviour to the potential cause. The NDB model provides a helpful philosophy when implementing person-centred care, as it considers the behaviour from the perspective of the person with dementia, rather than the caregiver. Additionally, the NDB model suggests behaviours occur due to the interaction between biological factors caused by the dementia and external factors such as the environment. Whilst the biological factors remain fixed, external factors such as the environment can be modified. For example, providing meaningful activity for the person with dementia may prevent some of the more difficult behaviour that caregivers struggle to manage (Volicer and Hurley, 2003). Being in an unfamiliar environment such as a hospital, with unfamiliar routines, could also create confusion and distress that may be displayed as agitation and possibly aggression. Most hospitals still do not have a system to identify whether a person has dementia, nor do they collect sufficient personal information to help with the support of specific behaviours associated with dementia. Futhermore, most hospitals do not have systems to aid communication or identify situations that may cause or exacerbate stress in this client group (Royal College of Psychiatrists, 2013).

If we are to improve the situation for people with dementia in acute contexts, sharing personal information with all staff but especially direct care staff could make a great difference in how staff perceive the behaviours of the person with dementia.

If we are to improve the situation for people with dementia in acute contexts, sharing personal information with all staff but especially direct care staff could make a great difference in how staff perceive the behaviours of the person with dementia. For example, understanding that an overhead spotlight may simulate a prisoner of war experience for a person with dementia could lead to altering the lighting is used for this person to reduce the likelihood of having antipsychotic medication prescribed. Other reasons for the behaviour should also be considered such as identifying if the person is in pain or if they are suffering from delirium.

Delirium is a treatable condition that causes short-term confusion and may be confused with symptoms similar to dementia. Delirium is thought to present in 8–17% of all older people presenting to an Emergency Department and 40% of those admitted to residential aged care (Inouye et al., 2014). The causes of delirium are multifactorial but often triggered by a physiological problem such as an infection, dehydration or constipation (Inouye et al., 2014). A Cochrane systematic review and meta-analysis demonstrated there was strong evidence for the effectiveness of multifactorial interventions in reducing the incidence and risk of delirium although only one study including people with dementia was located for this review (Siddiqi et al., 2016). When a person with dementia's behaviour changes from what is usual, this would be a clear signal for further investigations to ensure underlying conditions might be treated early.

It might be helpful at this point to return to Kitwood's five needs of a person with dementia (Figure 2.2) to explore how we might meet the emotional needs of the person with dementia. We all have emotional needs and it is often those closest to us that support us in meeting these needs. When a person with dementia requires a professionally led service, they may be isolated from those who provide comfort, the familiarity of routines and people who acknowledge their personal needs. Meeting the emotional needs of the person with dementia will then fall to the staff providing care. If staff do not see meeting the emotional needs of the person with dementia as their role, the person with dementia may then begin to display distressed behaviour as a result of unmet needs. It is often these behaviours that staff find challenging in any practice setting.

Comfort seeking behaviours may include the person with dementia seeking to hold another's hand; this may be the hands of other residents or staff members. When this need for comfort is not met, resulting distress could prompt a range of behaviours depending on the person involved. For example if a person with dementia is moved to a care home then they may not be used to sleeping alone and at night may consequently search for the person they usually share their bed with. This can be very problematic if the person with dementia is wandering into other residents' rooms and getting into another resident's bed. Viewing this behaviour as need-driven, i.e. a need for comfort, will aid understanding and so support staff in considering strategies that might provide that emotional attachment. An example of a strategy might be to make arrangements for the person's partner to sleep in the same room for a few nights to help the person settle into their new environment. In a small UK-based study I was involved in, family caregivers spoke about their continued need for intimacy with their loved one in spite of the dementia (Simpson et al., 2016). Providing the opportunity to sit on a couch together or even lie beside each other in a bed would support the person with dementia and their partner in meeting these ongoing needs (Bauer et al., 2013a; Simpson et al., 2016). Unfortunately, sexual expression is not always something that staff in residential aged care feel comfortable with and such discomfort may lead to staff labelling sexual relationships as aberrant behaviour (Simpson et al., 2015). There may also be older people who don't feel sexuality is relevant to them anymore (Simpson et al., 2016). The lack of acknowledgement that older people including those with dementia continue to have an interest in sex and/or intimacy may also have ramifications for people with dementia who identify as Lesbian, Gay, Bisexual, Transgender and Inter-Sex (LGBTI). Intimate relationships are particularly significant in the lives of LGBTI individuals due to previous rejection by families and wider experience of homophobia (Barrett et al., 2014). The assumption of heterosexuality in care services is often a barrier to older people and those with dementia from disclosing their sexuality. Understanding the collective history of the LGBTI community alongside the importance of gender identity are valuable first steps in appreciating the dilemma of disclosure (Barrett et al., 2015). LGBTI people feel it should be their decision to disclose their gender and/or sexuality but would value staff being open to these discussions (Barrett et al., 2014).

People with dementia may not be able to express their ongoing needs for sex, intimacy and comfort, so it is vital that health and care services support people irrespective of gender, sexuality or culture in addressing these needs in the way the person with dementia would wish. Practice scenario 7.1 provides an opportunity to consider how we might improve this aspect of care.

Practice scenario 7.1

A Care Home Manager recounted how staff were alerted when two residents, a gentleman and lady, both with dementia, were seen to be in the same room in states of undress. Both had removed their clothing: the gentleman from the waist down and the woman from the waist up. Staff were concerned whether the woman was able to consent as the gentleman often exhibited sexually disinhibited behaviour. Staff entered the room and separated the couple to find out from the woman if she was consenting to this encounter. When asked if she was OK, the woman told the Manager that this gentleman reminded her of her late husband and she was very happy to be in this condition with him. The staff then relaxed as it was deemed consensual. However, the Care Home Manager reflected that retrospectively there might have been a better way of handling this situation.

Source: unpublished data from Focus Groups, Simpson et al. (2016).

The situation in Practice scenario 7.1 may be further complicated if either of the residents were to have a surviving partner that lived externally to the care home. Surviving partners along with adult children of residents may feel discomfited when they witness their loved one embarking on a new relationship. Older people themselves in residential aged care have suggested their relationships should remain private and not necessarily be discussed with their families (Bauer et al., 2013a), although the families would not necessarily agree with this (Bauer et al., 2014b). Adopting a relationship-centred approach at such a point might be helpful to ensure everyone's needs are considered in a way that does not prevent the person with dementia from their right to sexual expression.

The situation of consensual sexual relationships is very different to sexual disinhibition, which means that the person with dementia is not able to control this behaviour. Disinhibition generally is a result of impaired judgement, lack of awareness of the effect of the behaviour on those around them and inability to edit impulsive behaviour. Sexual disinhibition is particularly rare in dementia and may be due to frontal lobe damage, delirium, a cerebral event or as a result of psychosis (Burns et al., 2012). Differentiating between need-driven behaviour and disinhibition is vital to support the wellbeing of the person with dementia and those around them. A full assessment to address sexual disinhibition and the associated risks for those who may be affected by the behaviour is required.

As an example, older female caregivers living in the community may be particularly vulnerable to repeated requests for sexual intercourse, sexual aggression or rape from their husbands and immediate support should be provided. There is limited research in the management of sexual disinhibition, although it is suggested that all cases be managed on a case-by-case basis and interventions should avoid responses resulting in humiliation or shame (Burns et al., 2012).

Activity 7. 2 Critical Thinking

Look at the time line you completed with the person with dementia in Activity 7.1.

Identify different behaviours over the course of the day this person might engage in – if you are having difficulty in thinking of any refer to Table 7.1.

Using the Need-Driven Dementia-Compromised Behaviour Model (NDB) and Kitwood's five needs of a person with dementia (Figure 2.2) what do you think this person is trying to communicate? Are there any times when there might be emotional needs not being met?

Consider the information from Practice scenario 7.1 and the preceding section: how might you develop a process for addressing these needs when an assessment of capacity is required?

Now we are going to consider a second model of considering behaviours of the person with dementia, the Progressively Lowered Stress Threshold Model, which considers how the external environment may be interacting with the inner world of the person with dementia. The Progressively Lowered Stress Threshold Model posits that a person with dementia has less ability to use environmental cues as the disease process continues and so requires the environment to be modified to accommodate the stress this causes (Smith et al., 2004). The focus of this model is the person–environment fit/interaction in modifying stress inducing triggers to reduce discomforting behaviours. External environmental demands such as noise or internal environmental demands such as pain may exceed the person with dementia's ability to adapt and cope. This ability to adapt and cope with external demands reduces as the dementia progresses. This means that people with dementia begin to develop anxious behaviours, which then progress to dysfunctional behaviour as the stressors accumulate. Therefore understanding how the person with dementia responds to the environment supports caregivers to make modifications to improve behaviour, a positive effect of which has been demonstrated in a number of studies (Gerdner et al., 2002; Huang et al., 2003).

Lyn Chenoweth and colleagues developed an intervention focusing on the person–environment fit (Chenoweth et al., 2014). This team developed and implemented a person-centred environment (PCE) intervention alongside a person-centred care (PCC) intervention, and also combined the two approaches (PCE+PCC). PCE, PCC and PCE+PCC were then compared to usual care. PCE and PCC in isolation improved agitation but improvement in the other outcomes (depression and quality of life) were not demonstrated. These results highlight the complexity of mapping behaviours to implementation of person-centred care and person-centred environmental changes.

Wendy Moyle and colleagues (2013b) developed the Capability Model of Dementia Care (CMDC) in Australia and found that staff showed more interest in understanding the behaviours of the person with dementia in relation to their biography. Based on the principles of person-centred and relationship-centred care, CMDC recognised the capabilities of the person with dementia and provided staff with clear guidance in how to use this knowledge of the person in an individualised care planning cycle. Implementation of the CMDC resulted in improved relationships between staff, residents and families with which came a greater understanding of the role biography played in the behaviours of the person with dementia (Moyle et al., 2013b). These qualitative findings were underpinned by later quantitative findings demonstrating that implementation of CMDC improved care staff attitudes towards, and experiences of, working and caring for the person with dementia (Moyle et al., 2016). Improving the relationships between care staff and people with dementia would seem to be a critical factor in reducing stress from the social environment for the person with dementia. Practice scenario 7.2 outlines staff training for the implementation of CMDC.

Practice scenario 7.2

Staff training in residential aged care (Cooke et al., 2014; Moyle et al., 2016) in the Capability Model of Dementia Care

Staff training comprises six, 2-hour face-to-face small group workshops covering the following areas:

- Dementia, values, and personhood
- Capabilities Model of Dementia Care: Care cycle, strengths and relationship-centred care capabilities: Feeling Valued & Play
- Communication: Care cycle – planning opportunities capabilities: Emotions & Senses, Imagination & Thought
- The care cycle: Facilitating care needs capabilities: Optimal Health & Sense of Control
- Morals, reflective practice capabilities: Case Review & Evaluation
- Mentor's role capabilities: Connection, Contribution & Natural World

We have now reviewed two models that support us in understanding why people with dementia may display behaviours that staff and family caregivers find challenging. However, it can sometimes be difficult to pinpoint the different triggers either within the person with dementia or within the environment that may give rise to these behaviours. A further approach to supporting the person with dementia and family caregivers in understanding and managing behaviours is the Activator–Behaviour–Consequence (ABC) model. Based on behavioural and social learning theory, the ABC model provides structured guidance to caregivers in how to assess and modify the context of behaviour (Logsdon et al., 2005; Teri et al., 2012). The ABC model has been used in a range of studies known as the Seattle Protocols wherein caregivers were taught problem-solving techniques using the ABC strategy as well as strategies to increase behavioural activation (pleasant events, exercise) (Teri et al., 1997, 2003, 2005, 2012). These studies demonstrated a reduction in behaviours and improved functioning. Additionally, Teri et al. (2005) also demonstrated benefits for caregivers in the community (reduced burden, increased quality of life and improved sleep) along with delayed institutionalisation when compared to those not using the Seattle Protocol. The key feature across these studies is a problem-solving and behavioural-activation approach delivered by trained clinicians enabling staff to understand the context of behaviour and ultimately anticipate potential difficulties. These strategies are also able to be used by Registered Nurses to identify if changes to the physical and social environment might reduce behaviours that staff or family caregivers may find difficult to cope with.

Practice scenario 7. 3

In a Practice Development workshop in a Tertiary Mental Health Centre, Edward was described as taking up a lot of staff time at lunchtime as he was always aggressive. Staff were prompted to use the ABC approach and identified the following information:

Activator: Lunchtime in the communal dining room.

Behaviour: Edward became aggressive towards other residents.

Consequence: Staff would need to have one person to sit with Edward to calm him down for one hour after lunch.

Biographical information: Speaking to his friend, staff were told that Edward was a very private person and did not like people coming to his flat. He would be rude to people and ask them to leave.

Change in practice: Staff arranged for Edward to have his lunch before everyone else came to the lunch room. Edward ate well without becoming aggressive and was then taken to a quiet corner where he was content to sit by himself.

Practice scenario 7.3 demonstrates the importance of knowing the person and their personality before dementia, as well as understanding the current context from the perspective of the person with dementia. This biographical knowledge then enables staff to anticipate that some situations will be stressful for some people and then to initiate a change to the way care is delivered or to adapt the social environment. Whilst this is important from an individual person's perspective, it becomes even more important when delivering person-centred care to a group of people (Brown Wilson and Davies, 2009).

Activity 7.3 Critical Thinking

Consider the information from Activity 7.1 and 7.2 and complete the following:

- Describe the behaviour – include how often it happens, when it happens, who is involved, the intensity of the behaviour and where it occurs.
- How does the personal information from Activity 7.1 influence this behaviour?
- How does the role of the caregiver influence this behaviour?
- How does the physical and social environment influence this behaviour?
- Are there medications that might be influencing this behaviour?

Now you have conducted an in-depth assessment on the behaviour, consider how you might address the behaviour using the ABC method below:

- What are the Activators that led to this Behaviour?
- What were the Behaviours that resulted?
- What are the Consequences for the person with dementia and staff?

From this process, identify different practices that could be implemented to improve the experience of the person with dementia and so reduce these behaviours. There are a range of resources at the end of this chapter that you can use to identify potential solutions.

The ABC approach has been successfully used in community environments (Teri et al., 1997, 2003, 2005, 2012) and may also be a useful tool to support staff in busy hospital wards in reassessing responses when dealing with behaviours exhibited by the person with dementia (Moyle et al., 2008). The incidence of people with dementia admitted to acute care settings is high and expected to rise (Travers et al., 2012). Interview studies with nurses caring for people with dementia in acute settings identify issues such as dealing with disruptive and aggressive behaviours including the use of chemical and physical restraint (Borbasi et al., 2006; Nolan, 2006; Moyle et al., 2011). A recent survey of UK hospitals showed that 61% of hospitals have a protocol for dealing with aggressive, violent or challenging behaviour and overall, the rate of antipsychotic prescriptions are falling (Royal College of Psychiatrists, 2013). While there may be times when antipsychotic medication may be needed, this should always be a last resort with strict protocols being followed. Adopting the ABC approach may be one way of addressing the primarily negative outcomes that people with dementia still experience when admitted to acute settings (Dewing and Dijk, 2016).

Meaningful care in the acute context requires respectful connections with the person with dementia that is facilitated by working with family caregivers (Nolan, 2006). Davina Porock and colleagues (Gladman et al., 2012; Clissett et al., 2013a, 2013b; Porock et al., 2015) explored the experience of hospitalisation from the perspective of the person with dementia, staff, family caregivers and co-patients in the UK. The disruption to normal routine was a core problem with behaviours seen as an attempt to regain a sense of control (Porock et al., 2015). Regaining a sense of control was achieved in different ways: meaningful activity such as organising belongings, distressed, agitated or aggressive behaviour or withdrawal (Porock et al., 2015).

Family caregivers similarly tried to gain a sense of control engaging in a range of strategies including monitoring the quality of care, complaining and questioning, gaining expertise, strategising, seeking support and taking advantage of the time in hospital to get things organised in the community. Family caregivers also attempted to give a sense of control to others such as the person with dementia, co-patients and staff. Such attempts included engaging the person with dementia in meaningful activity, helping out with care of the person with dementia and supporting co-patients to reduce the pressure on the nursing staff (Porock et al., 2015). A set of complex interactions occur within the disruption of hospital admission between the person with dementia, co-patients, family caregivers and staff. The behaviours exhibited by the person with dementia are in response to this disruption but may challenge staff. When this occurs, the relationship between all parties becomes disrupted and the focus of healthcare professionals is on trying to regain control rather than focusing on the person with dementia. Staff managed this disruption by seeking to protect themselves from the stressors of caring by suspending the personhood of the person with dementia (Clissett et al., 2013a). When staff responded to the disruption in this way, a common theme was their limited communication with the person with dementia even when there were opportunities to interact positively (Clissett et al., 2013a).

A focus on developing relationships is essential to implementing person-centred care in an acute setting (Nolan, 2006; Edvardsson and Nay, 2009; Clissett et al., 2013b). Clissett et al. (2013b) observed how staff promoted person-centred care in their interactions with the person with dementia, acknowledging the importance of existing relationships by including the person with dementia in decision-making and creating an inclusive environment (Clissett et al., 2013b). However, Clissett et al. (2013b) also observed how staff missed opportunities to promote person-centred care such as in the provision of a personalised environment that promotes a sense of identity and can provide prompts for staff to interact with the person with dementia (Edvardsson and Nay, 2009; Brown Wilson et al., 2013). Opportunities for involving people with dementia in activity were observed but rarely acted on by staff. Clissett et al. (2013b) concluded that this lack of staff involvement in activity may have contributed to disruptive behaviour as the person with dementia looked to find something meaningful to do.

Seeing the needs of the person with dementia as different from those of patients in an acute ward and subsequently prioritising care for others over the person with dementia leads to suspending the personhood of that person (Moyle et al., 2008; Clissett et al., 2013a). This may be attributed to the culture of care across acute settings that focuses on the task rather than the care with which it is delivered (Borbasi et al., 2006; Moyle et al., 2008; Dewing and Dijk, 2016). However, in a small qualitative study, ward staff identified that having a patient information pack supported them in knowing the person (Chater and Hughes, 2012). Further suggestions to improve care included recognising the importance of relationships; using handovers more effectively; and learning from each other, nurturing a team approach (Chater and Hughes, 2012). Furthermore, staff with positive attitudes towards people with dementia are more likely to have undertaken specific dementia education and identify higher levels of self-confidence in caring for a person with dementia (Travers et al., 2013). A tailored intervention for the acute care setting is outlined in Practice scenario 7.4.

Practice scenario 7.4

Dementia skills training for the acute sector (Nayton et al., 2014) – 'The view from here: skills in dementia care for acute settings'

Aims

- To increase staff awareness in how people with dementia experience the acute setting.
- To provide staff with an evidence-based assessment and observation techniques to understand the experience of the person with dementia.

Components

- Neurobiology and Person-centred Care;
- Communication Strategies;
- Information Gathering and Bedside Tests;
- Approaches to Pain Assessment;
- Activities for the Inpatient Setting;
- Behavioural Observation and Pharmacology;
- The Acute Care Environment.

The 25-minute micro teaching sessions were delivered by a Clinical Nurse Consultant (CNC) with specialist knowledge in dementia and delirium and extensive clinical experience of working with people with dementia in acute care settings. Staff were encouraged to identify how they might implement the information and sessions were delivered four times to maximise staff attendance. Dementia Champions were identified on each participating ward. A sustainability workshop was delivered on completion of the programme to identify ongoing strategies that could be embedded on the ward and included senior management.

The education programme above demonstrates an important starting point for managing behaviours that enable staff to understand the nature of dementia alongside the experience of the person with dementia. Earlier in the chapter, we reviewed Wendy Moyle's Capability Model of Dementia Care (Moyle et al., 2016), which supported staff in thinking differently. Both of these programmes require expert input and guidance and substantial support from the management. I have also been involved with staff in facilitating a change in practice in a less structured way (Practice scenario 7.5). This approach has not been rigorously tested but provides a good starting point to encourage staff to think differently about their care (Brown Wilson et al., 2013).

Practice scenario 7.5

Practice development in a tertiary environment

I was approached by an organisation that had been trained by the Bradford Dementia Group in person-centred care. Staff were struggling to identify how they could implement a change in practice and needed a more applied practice development approach rather than education. Adopting a facilitated approach, we used a case-based methodology where staff would bring a 'case' of a person with dementia who was exhibiting behaviour that staff found challenging. Each week the 'case' would be discussed in respect to the following framework:

- Knowing ourselves – how are staff responding to the behaviour of the person with dementia?
- Knowing the person – why might the person be responding in this way, given the biographical details known about the person?
- Developing person-centred goals with the family using biographical information the family shared.
- Developing a plan of care anticipating the needs of the person with dementia.
- Developing shared understandings – communication strategies with staff and families to promote the sharing of personal information that enables person-centred care using the following format:

Domain of PCC	**Capturing the evidence**
Finding out what matters to the person	Knowing the person – biography
Knowing why the routine is significant	Biography – involving the family
Attention to details	Planning the care
Adopting a consistent approach that values the person	Handover and/or ward-based communication e.g. huddles

Educational interventions have also been developed for families, primarily in residential aged care environments. Such an example is the Family Involvement in Care (FIC) intervention (Maas et al., 2004) that was developed to improve family caregivers' experience of special care dementia units. This involved education of the caregiver about the trajectory of the dementia and how it might impact on their loved one, alongside preparation for partnership with staff, which included negotiation of care (Maas et al., 2004). The underpinning theory behind this intervention was that the interface between staff and family caregiver influenced the 'person–environment fit' for the person with dementia. We will revisit partnerships with caregivers in the following chapter. Returning now to our organisational approach in developing relationship-based approaches to care use the following activity to develop an educational strategy for the area in which you practice.

Activity 7.4 Reflection

Using the following table develop an educational strategy for practice.

Identify the strategies that would facilitate an evidence-based education strategy at each level of an organisation. Identify the people you would include and the anticipated outcomes you would expect:

Level of the organisation	Staff involved	Educational strategy	Anticipated outcome
Macro level	e.g. Senior management	e.g. Awareness raising	e.g. Agreement to fund training
Meso level	e.g. Unit manager		e.g. Reduction in adverse events
Micro level Direct care	e.g. Nurses and allied health care		e.g. Improvement in management of behaviour
Micro level Direct care	e.g. Person with dementia and family caregivers		e.g. Improved communication

Conclusion

In residential environments living in a community of people also poses challenges for the person with dementia as they have to navigate a perpetually unfamiliar environment, routines they have no control over and constantly meeting unfamiliar people. Making sense of what the range of behaviours mean for different people, and how they come to express distress, pain or discomfort is integral to good quality person-centred care. The discussion in this chapter has demonstrated the value of understanding the impact of personal and social environment on the person with dementia. A key aspect of this is the anticipation of what is needed to avoid unnecessary stress being experienced by the person with dementia within the social environment. The use of the ABC approach provides a structure staff can use to avoid stressful situations that adversely impact the person with dementia. Understanding the perspective of the person with dementia is integral to seeing behaviours as a mechanism of communication. Staff need to be supported in the development of personal and respectful communication leading to positive relationships that then enable a person-centred approach to care. This is not something that happens by chance but needs to be actively facilitated through education and support at all levels of the organisation.

Final reflections

In the previous chapter, we considered the structural issues within organisations that facilitated relationship-based approaches to care with a focus on the physical environment. This focus demonstrated some of the issues with person–environment fit. In this chapter, we have considered the perspective of the person with dementia and how the social environment impacts on their behaviour. We have examined a number of interventions to support us in viewing behaviour as communication to enable the implementation of relationship-based approaches to care. The next chapter will focus on supporting and developing partnerships with caregivers, the next stage in developing relationship-based approaches to care.

Further reading

DBMAS

Dementia Behaviours Management Advisory Service (DBMAS) is an Australian Government initiative. This service provides individualised support for family caregivers who are supporting a person with dementia with rapidly changing behavioural and psychological needs that are negatively influencing the person with dementia's care and Quality of Life. DBMAS also provides resources for professionals. Available at: http://dbmas.org.au/resources/library/ (accessed 27/01/17).

Dealing with Behaviours of People with Dementia: A Guide for Family Carers. Available at: http://dbmas.org.au/uploads/resources/A_Guide_for_Family_Carers.pdf (accessed 27/01/17).

DMAS BPSD app – this app is available to download via Google Play or the app store, providing a ready reference guide on your phone to a range of behaviours with suggested management techniques. This can be used by family and professional caregivers. Available at: http://dbmas.org.au/resources/bpsd-guide-app/ (accessed 27/01/17).

Beyond Blue

This organisation provides mental health advice and support to everyone in Australia regardless of who they are or where they live. Beyond Blue commissioned a systematic review on the evidence of supporting older people with mental health issues in the community and residential environments. They produced the booklet:'What works to promote emotional wellbeing in older people: a guide for aged care staff working in community or residential care settings', which covers a range of interventions that can be used to promote emotional wellbeing or to help people with anxiety or depression. It summarises the strength of evidence for each intervention and gives case studies to show how the interventions have been used with older people. Available at: http://resources.beyondblue.org.au/prism/file?token=BL/1263A (accessed 27/01/17).

Supporting sexual expression resources

Sexuality Assessment Tool (SexAT) has been developed by researchers (Bauer et al., 2013b and 2014a) for residential aged care facilities using the evidence base alongside expert and peer opinion. This encourages an organisational approach by considering policies, education and training for residents, families and staff and assessing how sexuality is managed in direct care. Available at: www.agedcare.org.au/publications/agendas-docs-images/sexuality-assessment-tool-sexat-for-residential-aged-care-facilities (accessed 27/01/17).

Supporting LGBTI people living with dementia

The following website provides video stories of LGBTI people speaking about their experiences of dementia: www.fightdementia.org.au/about-dementa/resources/lgbti (accessed 27/01/17).

Val's Café

Val's Café was established in 2009, as a project seeking to improve the health and wellbeing of older lesbian, gay, bisexual, trans and intersex (LGBTI) people. Central to this aim is creating safe and inclusive services that recognise and value older LGBTI people. This is achieved by working directly with service providers to foster an understanding of the unique histories and experiences of older LGBTI people. See: www.valscafe.org.au/ (accessed 27/01/17).

Working Therapeutically with LGBTI Clients: A Practice Wisdom Resource
This is a general guide to working with LGBTI clients aimed at counselling but provides relevant background knowledge for all practitioners. Available at: www.lgbtihealth.org.au/sites/default/files/practice-wisdom-guide-online.pdf (accessed 27/01/17).

8

Supporting the families of people living with dementia

Learning objectives

By the end of this chapter, the reader will be able to:

- Explore the meaning of caregiving in dementia from the family's perspective.
- Examine the support that family caregivers say they need to care for the person with dementia.
- Critically evaluate the effectiveness of interventions that support family caregivers.
- Develop a plan for healthcare professionals such as nurses to work in partnership with family caregivers.

Introduction

In Chapter 4 we discussed how interactions between families and staff could promote relationship-based approaches to care and enhance a biographical approach to care planning at the micro level of the organisation. That discussion was focused primarily on how families were contributing to the support of a person with dementia when in a residential environment. We know that most people with dementia live in the community and that family caregivers and other supporters are essential in enabling a person with dementia to remain living in their community. This means that the wellbeing of family caregivers is being increasingly recognised as vital to the ability of people living with dementia to remain living at home.

The support provided by family caregivers in dementia care is recognised worldwide as an essential resource, and one that is to be valued (Wimo and Prince, 2010). However, we also know that dementia caregivers have generally worse health outcomes than non-dementia caregivers (Pinquart and Sorenson, 2004), experiencing a higher rate of burden, distress and poor health (Brodaty and Donkin, 2009). This information has been known for some time and governments across the world are developing strategies to address the support of caregivers. For example, some Western countries have implemented national guidelines through Acts of Parliament; see for example the The Care Act, 2014 (England only) (Department of Health, 2013) and the Carer Recognition Act, 2010 (Commonwealth of Australia, 2011). Such strategies then guide how services are organised (at both the macro and meso levels of organisations) and delivered (micro level of organisations). For instance, a range of day and residential respite services exist internationally to support caregivers in maintaining their caregiving role (Naville et al., 2015). Despite this, caregivers to people living with dementia routinely speak about the difficulties they encounter in locating or engaging with services that meet their needs.

Many of the families I have spoken with describe their journey through dementia caregiving as a rollercoaster as they attempt to navigate the many services and systems experiencing limited or fragmented support. Each family caregiver will have an individual narrative of how they began their dementia journey and why they undertook the caregiving role. Each caregiver will also have a personal history that shapes their relationship with the person they are caring for, the degree of social support they have access to and what caregiving means for them. The nature of the caregiving journey will influence whether family caregivers experience positive aspects of caregiving, referred to as 'uplifts' or a sense of burden or psychological distress. We have discussed throughout this book the value of relationships, and relationships between the caregiver, the person with dementia and wider family members are equally important. Wider family relationships are not something we may ordinarily consider within nursing practice but in focusing on relationship-based approaches to dementia care, family relationships are another aspect we need to consider as we support family caregivers, especially in the community. In Chapter 7 we discussed how we as professionals could influence the social environment, which may be more problematic when we are in a person's own home. Therefore in this chapter, we will consider caregivers' experience of caregiving and examine how organisations might use this knowledge to support caregivers more effectively. We will apply this information to our day-to-day practice with family caregivers and examine how we might engage in partnership working with families.

What shapes the experience of dementia caregiving for families?

Caregiving is a complex process. Healthcare professionals tend to understand caregiving as providing instrumental support to the person with dementia. However in speaking with many caregivers over the years throughout my practice and research roles, I have found that the experience of caregiving is shaped by many factors, including the dyadic relationship of the caregiver and care recipient. Healthcare professionals such as nurses tend to come into contact with caregivers once they require professional services with the reasons why such support was needed often remaining unexplored. Not recognising the underlying issues affecting the family caregiver that triggered service involvement may account for the ongoing concerns raised by caregivers that the resources, information and support being provided do not meet their needs. To deliver person-centred and relationship-centred care with caregivers as active contributors we need to consider the broader level of the caregiving experience.

It is without doubt that caregiving creates stress and burden for family caregivers. Certainly, caregivers of people living with dementia report higher levels of psychological distress and burden when compared to those caring for a person with a physical disability or with non-caregivers (Pinquart and Sorenson, 2003).This level of distress may be the reason support services are initially sought out and may explain why the research has focused almost exclusively on the alleviation of distress to enable continued caregiving. Pearlin and colleagues' (1990) process model has been widely accepted in identifying the components of caregiver stress and is often used to consider outcomes of interventions. Pearlin et al. (1990) suggest that the background of caregivers along with stressors that relate to themselves, their wider lives and the person they are caring for influence the outcomes they experience with social support and coping mechanisms mediating these outcomes. Further work by Pinquart and Sorenson (2004) explored how positive affect, quality of life and life satisfaction were related to both stressors and uplifts of the caregiving experience, impacting on Subjective Well-Being of the caregiver (see Figure 8.1).

Using the model in Figure 8.1 provides an opportunity to explore how relationships between the background, environment and different experiences of the caregiver may influence the outcomes caregivers experience. Appreciating the caregivers' personal experience of caregiving will support us as professionals in developing strategies to work with the caregiver more effectively. Social support and coping mechanisms can buffer some of the psychological distress or burden experienced by caregivers. This is key information for nurses and other healthcare professionals to ensure we don't destabilise established mechanisms for coping and social support already in place. There may also be times when social support for caregivers might

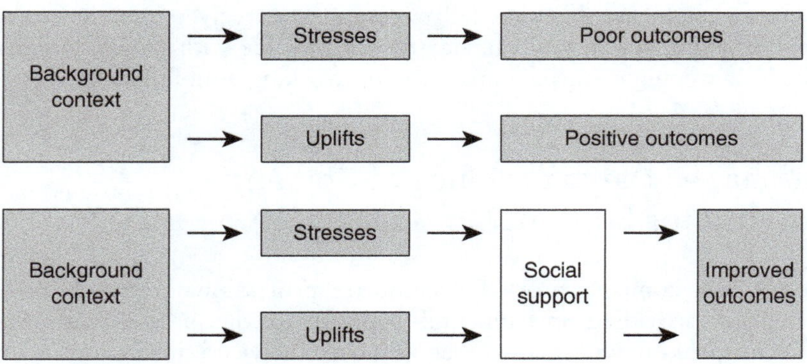

Figure 8.1 Model of caregiving

Based on Pearlin et al. (1990) and Pinquart and Sorenson (2004)

be integrated into a range of easily accessible services to enhance caregivers' coping strategies. Successfully identifying this hidden aspect of service delivery will enable professionals to support caregivers more effectively. To begin this process, complete Activity 8.1 to identify the key stressors and positive experiences you have observed in your work with caregivers.

Activity 8.1 Reflection

In your experience of supporting people with dementia and their family caregivers, identify some of the key stressors caregivers may experience and the positive experiences they have shared with the person with dementia and how these have contributed to the caregiver's subjective wellbeing. We will be building on this activity as we progress through this chapter.

	Impact on the caregiver: the professional perspective	**Impact on the caregiver: the caregiver perspective – see Activity 8.2 to complete this column**
Key stressors:		
Positive experiences:		

There are some factors that are influenced by the social determinants of health that shape a caregiver's experience of caregiving. We know that economic and social disadvantage adversely affects the available personal, social and financial resources people have to draw on. For instance, being an ethnic minority caregiver in any given country is perceived to create a double jeopardy due to economic and social disadvantage, which often limits the choices caregivers have and how they interact with services. There is also the common perception that there exists greater familial support in some cultures, which is not always the case. For example, globalisation now means many families are living in geographically distant places. Of course, this is not to say that all cultural groups perceive caregiving in the same way. In large studies conducted in the USA, Sorenson and Pinquart (2005) found distinct differences between the experience of caregiving between ethnic minority groups when compared to white caregivers (Pinquart and Sorenson, 2005). Those ethnic groups reporting better psychological health expressed pride in fulfilling filial or spousal responsibilities, enhanced closeness with a care receiver, and satisfaction with one's competence in relation to caregiving (Pinquart and Sorenson, 2005). Yet when looking across different ethnic groups, Sorenson and Pinquart (2005) concluded that the predictors of depression and health remained constant. The central message from this research is ensuring caregivers from ethnic minority groups have access to culturally responsive services and resources to address some of the disadvantage they experience. For example, more ethnic minority caregivers remain in employment and so need flexible times for services. Healthcare professionals must also be mindful of making the assumption that caregivers from differing cultural backgrounds have a greater level of familial support and so do not need formal services. Whilst we may be unable to alter the underlying disadvantage, as healthcare professionals we are in the position of being able to ensure appropriate and flexible access to services.

Caregiving continues to remain a gendered issue with notable differences in psychological health, physical health, and caregiving stressors between men and women (Pinquart and Sorenson, 2006b). Compared with male caregivers, females report longer hours of caring, increased frequency of problem behaviours, higher levels of burden, poorer physical health and lower levels of wellbeing (Pinquart and Sorenson, 2006b). Nevertheless, there is now a changing social context with more women in the workforce and an increasing number of men supporting caregiving. When the experience of male caregivers is examined, similar issues to women are reported (Pinquart and Sorenson, 2006b). This suggests that interventions targeted at relieving some of the caregiving stressors experienced by women such as getting help with Activities of Daily Living (ADL) assistance and support for current and previous relational stressors, might in fact benefit all caregivers.

The experience of caregiving is also diverse when considering family relationships and who is involved in the caregiving. Being an adult child of a person living with dementia will affect the caregiving experience differently to a husband, wife or partner (referred to as spouses). Although the tasks of caring provided by adult children and children-in-law are comparable to those of spouses, spousal caregivers report poorer physical health, and more depressive symptoms than adult children or children-in-law caregivers (Pinquart and Sorenson, 2011). This may be because spousal caregivers are living with the person with dementia, providing more hours of care. Irrespective of the relationship, the same level of burden and positive aspects of caregiving are experienced. However the largest predictors of psychological distress across all types of caregivers remain physical health and levels of informal support (Pinquart and Sorenson, 2011). From this, we might infer that interventions aimed at improving physical health and promoting informal support could support all caregivers. To fully appreciate the caregiving experience we need to hear the stories caregivers share with us. Using Activity 8.2 develop the table started in Activity 8.1 to see how the information you identified may or may not be reflected in the stories shared by caregivers.

Activity 8.2 Reflection

Consider the family caregiver from Activity 8.1 and answer the following questions:

- How did this caregiver talk about their experience of caregiving?
- How did the caregiver speak about their health?
- How did where the person with dementia and their caregiver live influence their experience?
- How did the caregiver describe their relationship with the person with dementia?

Returning to the table started in Activity 8.1, complete the second column: Impact on the caregiver: the caregiver perspective – were these areas stressors or positive experiences?

Now consider how this information differed or was similar to the professional perspective. What does this mean for the services being provided to this family caregiver?

Caregivers' perception of caring is an important factor in considering the type of support that might be helpful for family caregivers. One study has demonstrated that spousal caregivers report caregiving as an opportunity to reciprocate or an extension of their marital relationship whilst adult child caregivers saw caregiving as providing opportunities for personal growth and development (Lloyd et al., 2014). There is also a growing body of research on the positive nature of caring, described as 'uplifts' or gains, from the caregiving itself or from the dynamic between caregiver and the person with dementia (Brodaty and Donkin, 2009; Carbonneau et al., 2010; Lloyd et al., 2014).

Interestingly, two meta-analyses suggest that caregiver wellbeing and caregiver burden are influenced by different factors (Pinquart and Sorenson, 2003, 2004). Pinquart and Sorenson (2004) identify that subjective wellbeing is influenced by positive events whereas burden or depression is primarily influenced by negative events. This means that experiencing positive events with the care recipient or enabling caregivers to continue with activities they enjoy may increase caregiver wellbeing. Caregiving stressors have a greater impact on depression and don't appear to impact on wellbeing in the same way. This means that the caregiver's experience of subjective wellbeing can be protected even when caregiving stressors exist. At a practice level, providing time for caregivers to do things that give their life meaning could be a more effective way to improve subjective wellbeing rather than trying to remove caregiving stressors. We do need to recognise that the growing level of impairment of the person with dementia will have a negative impact on caregiver wellbeing (Pinquart and Sorenson, 2004). From a service delivery perspective, we need to consider how these impairments alter the caregiver's experience of the uplifts or gains they perceive from caregiving. Therefore in our practice we might support the family caregiver in developing skills to manage behaviours associated with greater impairment in dementia thus contributing to self-efficacy, which has a significant, positive association with positive aspects of caregiving (Semiatin and O'Connor, 2012).

Practice scenario 8.1

Art and Dementia Programme

The National Gallery of Australia have implemented an Art and Dementia Programme similar to the one run by the Museum of Modern Art (MoMA) in New York. People with dementia and their caregivers are supported by trained volunteers in small groups to

(Continued)

(Continued)

engage in conversation about the artwork. Initial evaluations suggest that the social interaction in a supportive environment enable the person with dementia and their caregiver to have a positive shared experience. In this context, the Art and Dementia Programme may provide a valuable focus for improving quality of life for the person with dementia and providing support to family caregivers.

Opportunities for the caregiver and person with dementia to experience positive events together are one way of promoting the positive impact of the caregiving experience (Carbonneau et al., 2010; Lloyd et al., 2014). Positive experiences in dementia caregiving are not automatic and may require the caregiver to actively create or consider opportunities for positive experiences (Lloyd et al., 2014). The positive nature of caregiving is also influenced by the quality of the relationship between the person with dementia and the caregiver (Nolan et al., 1996; Carbonneau et al., 2010). For instance, having a positive relationship with the person with dementia prior to a diagnosis is more likely to support the caregiver in identifying relationship gains (Lloyd et al., 2014). Caregivers themselves spoke about the need for acceptance and a positive attitude towards caregiving with some drawing on strengths such as faith or a supportive social network (Lloyd et al., 2014). Therefore, supporting caregivers in their family relationships and helping them to cognitively restructure their caregiving experience may also be helpful. However, not everyone starts with a positive relationship and so tailored support might be needed for the person with dementia and the caregiver to work on their relationship and to access support from the wider family (Drentea et al., 2006).

Activity 8.3 Reflection

1. Identify examples of positive experiences that might be available in your community for people living with dementia and their caregivers to enjoy.
2. What is it about these activities that might improve subjective wellbeing of the caregiver?
3. Are there other activities you could think of that would enable a person with dementia and their caregiver to enjoy time together?

This brings us to the more personal factors that might influence how caregivers experience caregiving. Lindauer and Harvath (2015) identified that caregivers perceived the changes in the person with dementia as both negative and positive. On the one hand, the disease process meant that the caregiver experienced concomitant losses, in the loss of the person they knew, the change to becoming a caregiver and the reduction of wider social support. However, caregivers also described opportunities for personal growth and of a positive nature within the opportunities to care (Lindauer and Harvath, 2015). There were similar themes derived from a critical review of qualitative studies considering the positive caregiver experience (Lloyd et al., 2014). In this paper, additional themes related to positive approaches to caregiving included feeling satisfaction in being in the role of caregiver, as well as the development of a sense of competence and mastery in providing care. Caregivers also described emotional rewards in giving care as well as relationship gains in spending time with the care recipient. Being able to fulfil a sense of duty was also expressed as well as the opportunity to give something positive back to the person they were caring for (Lloyd et al., 2014).

Practice scenario 8. 2

Dementia Adventure

Dementia Adventure is a UK not-for-profit organisation that provides supported opportunities for people with dementia and their caregivers to enjoy activities and the outdoors. Activities include:

- Walk and Talk Park tours which are operated in dementia accessible parks by volunteers providing a free opportunity for people with dementia to access nature.
- The design and delivery of short breaks and travel opportunities for people with dementia, their family and friends. This enables a supported holiday where new activities can be tried and caregivers can relax and enjoy the time with their loved one.

Understanding the experience and perspective of the caregiver provides a different lens from which we as healthcare professionals might now consider the range of support that might prove beneficial. When considering the caregivers' perspective, for those not able to see the positive gains of caregiving, we might need to explore how to alleviate the stressors they are experiencing. Alternatively, by strengthening the positive experiences there might be increased caregiver wellbeing that might enable them to cope better with the stressors they are experiencing. We will always be faced with situations we are unable to change and this approach may provide a clearer focus on the breadth of support available to the caregiver. Use Activity 8.4 to consider how this might be achieved in your practice.

Activity 8.4 Analysis

Using the table you have completed in Activity 8.1 and 8.2 within this chapter, identify examples of interventions/activities that might alleviate the stress or improve the positive experience for family caregivers.

(Continued)

(Continued)

	Impact on the caregiver	An example of an intervention you might consider to alleviate the stressor or protect/support the positive experience
Key stressors:		
Positive experiences:		

Compare what you have written to the model in Figure 8.1; how might these interventions support the subjective wellbeing of the family caregiver?

What interventions are effective for caregivers?

There has been a greater focus on providing non-pharmacological interventions for the person with dementia that now advocates providing caregiver support and education (Griffin et al., 2015). Caregiver interventions can be broadly grouped into: pyscho-educational interventions, counselling or supportive therapies, respite care, case management or multicomponent interventions (Pinquart and Sorenson, 2006a; Thompson et al., 2007; Parker et al., 2008; Olazarán et al., 2010; Schoenmakers et al., 2010). This section provides an overview of the systematic reviews and meta-analyses undertaken in this area of research to enable you to examine how the evidence might support your practice or the services you provide.

Pyscho-educational interventions generally refer to caregiver training focusing on knowledge, communication, skills and attitudes. Approaches adopted within these interventions may include problem-solving approaches for day-to-day caregiving issues, how to increase pleasant events, coping or self-management strategies conducted individually or in a group environment. The mode of delivery can be quite varied, ranging from providing information to caregivers as passive recipients to engaging caregivers in interactive strategies such as role plays. Overall, there is broad agreement in the literature that psycho-educational interventions are effective (Pinquart and Sorenson, 2006a; Thompson et al., 2007; Parker et al., 2008; Olazarán et al., 2010). Psycho-educational interventions have been found to be effective in a range of areas and for diverse reasons: Pinquart and Sorenson (2006a) found a greater positive effect size for interventions that involved the active participation of family caregivers in the intervention; Parker et al. (2008) found a small and immediate effect size for all psycho-educational interventions on caregiver depression and subjective wellbeing and Thompson et al. (2007) found an effect size for burden. In considering effects of caregiver education on the persons with dementia, Brodaty and Arasaratnam (2012) found that non-pharmacological interventions delivered by family caregivers were as effective as pharmacological interventions in reducing Behavioural and Psychological Disturbances (BPSD) for the person living with dementia.These findings are similar to studies implementing the Seattle Protocols that have been developed to support family caregivers in managing BPSD through targeted individualised, person-centred approaches (Teri et al., 2012). The Seattle Protocols (Practice scenario 8.3) have supported caregivers in reducing depression and subjective burden by supporting them in being less reactive to behavioural problems. Caregivers also report an improvement in the quality of life for the person with dementia when undertaking this intervention (Teri et al., 2005, 2012).

Practice scenario 8.3

Seattle Protocols (Teri et al., 2005, 2012)

Lind Teri and colleagues have developed a pyscho-educational intervention that recognises the person–environment fit and encourages family caregivers in identifying triggers that may prompt behavioural issues that caregivers find difficult to manage. The protocol focuses on current, observable interactions within the unique psychosocial context of caregiving.

This intervention comprises the following components:

1. Identify triggers using the Activator, Behaviour, Consequence (ABC) approach. Problem behaviours interfere with the ability of the caregiver to provide care and this decreases the person with dementia's enjoyment of life. Caregivers are asked to identify three behaviours they would like to change and rate these on how problematic they are and how often they occur. Strategies for changing the Activator or Consequences are discussed and a behaviour modification plan agreed.
2. Communication skills – supporting caregivers to communicate clearly and compassionately so as not to overload the person experiencing dementia.
3. Ways of increasing pleasant events are discussed.
4. Understanding dementia and developing realistic expectations.
5. Developing collaborative partnerships with all involved.

This intervention can be delivered by a range of professionals, including nurses who work with the family caregiver in implementing this approach. This intervention is delivered over eight weekly sessions with monthly telephone follow-ups for four months. This intervention has been developed and successfully delivered in a number of community environments.

Supportive and Counselling therapies are generally considered to include a more passive style of support through self-help in either groups or individual sessions. Brodaty and Donkin (2009) suggest that social support may provide a buffer against burden and distress although caution that unwanted social support may be more stressful than helpful. Thompson et al. (2007) concluded that interventions aimed at a more passive approach in supporting and/or providing information to carers of people with dementia were not uniformly effective. Parker et al. (2008) found a significant effect in group support although the studies used in the meta-analysis had small sample sizes and so these results need to be interpreted with caution.

The most extensive study on caregiver counselling and support is the New York University Caregiver Intervention (NYUCI) (Practice scenario 8.4). The family counselling sessions in this intervention were aimed at enabling caregivers to mobilise social support from within their network (Drentea et al., 2006). These sessions expanded the social support network for caregivers, increasing satisfaction with emotional support and practical assistance from family and friends (Roth et al., 2005). This level of satisfaction was attributed, in part, to having socially supportive contacts come into the home to provide emotional support and so providing psychological respite for the caregiver (Drentea et al., 2006). NYUCI also demonstrated significant positive effects on depressive symptoms of the caregiver for up to three years (Mittelman et al., 2004a), a positive impact on caregiver physical health (Mittelman et al., 2007) and significantly improved caregiver reaction to problem behaviours (Mittelman et al., 2004b). Furthermore NYUCI also significantly delayed admission into residential care (Mittelman et al., 2006) and was found to support the transition to institutionalisation when it occurred (Gaugler et al., 2008). As NYUCI was trialled over a 20-year period, it was also able to explore the impact on the caregiver following the death of the person they were caring for and found reduced depressive symptoms in the caregivers in the intervention group before and after bereavement. These findings suggest resilience in the intervention group that was not present in the control group (Haley et al., 2008).

Practice scenario 8.4

New York University Caregiver Intervention (NYUCI) (Mittelman et al., 2003)

This intervention was developed and tested by Mary Mittelman and colleagues using a large randomised controlled trial between 1987 and 2009. The intervention focused on counselling and support with the following components:

1. Six individual and family counselling sessions within the first four months:
    - An individual counselling session
    - Four family counselling sessions aimed at enabling caregivers to mobilise social support from within their network to encourage other family members to provide more concrete assistance with caregiving and emotional support
    - A second individual counselling session
2. Access to a support group over the course of the dementia journey.
3. Ad hoc counselling when requested by the caregiver or another family member.

This intervention has been developed and delivered by researchers in research environments and is now being replicated and rolled out to community services.

Respite or replacement care has been defined as something that provides the caregiver with a break, which can be internal or external (Neville et al., 2015) and depending on the country and region in which the caregiver lives, may take the form of day centres, in-home care, short periods of residential care, emergency replacement, support on holidays or short breaks, or the opportunity of the person with dementia to live in the home of the respite caregiver (known as Shared Lives).

Although respite or replacement care services are widely available, these services are often underutilised (Bruen and Howe, 2009; Neville et al., 2015). Equally the impact of respite for caregiver outcomes is mixed. Respite care was found to have a small but significant effect on caregiver depression, burden and subjective wellbeing by Pinquart and Sorenson (2006a). Yet a recent Cochrane Review found no significant effects on respite care compared to no respite care on any caregiver variables (Maayan et al., 2014). These differing findings may be due to the lack of choice or accessibility of services, the rigid nature of services and a lack of flexibility in how respite might be able to be used so making it difficult for caregivers to access support when they need it (Neville et al., 2015). Regarding residential respite care, caregivers have also raised concerns about the disorientation for the person with dementia and the ability of the service to cope with their complex needs (Neville et al., 2015). The underutilisation of services should be a key concern if we are endeavouring to meet the needs of caregivers throughout their dementia journey. A pertinent question for health professionals to consider is: are there the mechanisms for asking caregivers what they need and then is there a responsive or flexible system to deliver this? Considering flexible, cost-effective respite options for the family caregiver is a challenge for services that struggle with government funding priorities. That said, increasing pleasant events to support caregiver wellbeing might be one practical option as demonstrated by Practice scenario 8.5.

Practice scenario 8.5

Wellbeing day for family caregivers

One community service in the UK created a wellbeing day for caregivers as part of their respite service. Whilst the person with dementia was being cared for by the services, caregivers were able to drop in to a central location and have a health check with a Registered Nurse alongside pamper and wellbeing activities such as head massage, hand massage and manicure stations. Caregivers booked in for time slots and could spend as long or as little time as they wished. The evaluations were very positive with caregivers saying they felt revived and supported after this opportunity to focus on their own wellbeing.

Case management, although focused on the person with dementia, has a substantial role in providing support to the caregiver in accessing and managing formal care services. Although the role may vary between countries it generally involves assessment, planning and overseeing delivery of care and carer education (Reilly et al., 2015). Reilly et al. (2015) undertook a meta-analysis of case management on carer burden, quality of life and time to institutionalisation finding only small to moderate effect sizes across all outcomes. Other studies have found that family caregivers who do not live with the care recipient are more likely to act as case managers, accessing a range of different services to support the person they are caring for (Brodaty and Donkin, 2009).

The Admiral Nurse role in the UK has also been developed to support family caregivers of people living with dementia in the community. The Admiral Nurse provides a therapeutic relationship, undertakes a carer assessment, providing targeted information, skills training and education. There has been limited research to consider the effectiveness of this role although it has been evaluated positively by carers as providing focused support specifically for the needs of the caregiver (Bunn et al., 2016). However, it is unclear how Admiral Nurses work with other services and whether they improve carer outcomes when compared to other carer support provided in the community (Bunn et al., 2016).

Multicomponent interventions. A number of different components within an intervention are grouped as multicomponent interventions. As there may be a range of interventions being used, they can be problematic to compare. Olazarán et al. (2010) concluded that multicomponent caregiver education and support had a similar effect size to pharmacological treatment of the person with dementia in delaying institutionalisation, improving caregiver mood, physical wellbeing and quality of life. Pinquart and Sorenson (2006a) found that multicomponent interventions only influenced time to institutionalisation. A well known multicomponent intervention developed in the US is the Resources for Enhancing Alzheimer's Caregiver Health (REACH) studies. REACH was initially a multisite intervention designed to test out a number of interventions for caregivers based on each aspect of the stress–health model involving six sites with 1,222 caregivers and care recipients (Schulz et al., 2003; Belle et al., 2006). Standardised protocols and treatment manuals were developed ensuring fidelity of the interventions across sites so it was clear what the outcomes could be attributed to. It was evident from across the different sites that these interventions each produced improved yet different outcomes for the caregivers (Schulz et al., 2003). The findings from these independent studies were then combined into a single intervention known as REACH II. A key difference in the REACH II studies was the ethnic diversity of caregivers with equal numbers of White, African American and Hispanic ethnicities. The intervention (Practice scenario 8.6) included:

- Home environment assessment;
- Social support;
- Managing problem behaviours of the care recipient;
- Self-care behaviours such as managing one's health and stress management techniques.

The in-home component enables caregivers to identify and prioritise different behaviours with support for engaging the person with dementia in meaningful and pleasant activities tailored to the person with their abilities. This part of the intervention demonstrated significantly greater improvements in quality of life (as measured by indicators of depression, burden, social support, self-care, and patient problem behaviours) and a reduction in rates of clinical depression between the intervention and control groups. Institutionalisation of care recipients did not significantly differ, although rates of placement were higher in the control group than in the intervention group (Belle et al., 2006). Improvement was also seen in caregivers' self-perceived health within the intervention group suggesting that positive experience and satisfaction in caregiving may have health-enhancing effects (Basu et al., 2015).

Practice scenario 8.6

Resources for Enhancing Alzheimer's Caregiver Health (REACH) (Schulz et al., 2003)

This intervention was initially tested as six individual interventions and then combined into REACH II focusing on a tailored intervention for the caregiver of the person with dementia. The aim of this intervention is to reduce stress and burden for the caregiver whilst providing care within the home.

Components of the model include:

1. Individual information and support strategies such as caregiver self-care (e.g. relaxation techniques) and health behaviours.
2. Psycho-educational and Skill-Based Training Approaches to support behaviour management known as behaviour prescriptions.
3. Home-Based Environmental Interventions using home visits.
4. Group Support via phone.

The intervention was delivered via four to six therapeutic phone calls and home visits over a six-month period.

The REACH programme of research has seen the translation of an effective multi-centre trial for use by different community organisations and is now being developed internationally (Heinrich et al., 2014; Lykens et al., 2014; Cheung, et al., 2015). REACH II has also been modified for use by the Veterans Association (REACH-VA) (Nichols et al., 2011) and by community organisations (REACH-OUT) (Burgio et al., 2009).

Activity 8.5 Critical Thinking

Using the table you completed in Activity 8.4 how might you develop some of the interventions you identified to include the evidence base in the previous section?

(Continued)

(Continued)

	Impact on the caregiver	An example of an intervention you might consider to alleviate the stressor or protect/support the positive experience	How might this be developed using the evidence base reviewed?
Key stressors:			
Positive experiences:			

Developing partnership working with family caregivers

The interventions identified in the previous section have been developed and delivered by research teams and then adapted for use by community organisations. The ability to evaluate this evidence can contribute to the implementation of effective caregiver support strategies at a personal practice level as well as a service delivery level. In this section we will explore how we might use this evidence to implement a relationship-based approach to working with caregivers.

In Chapter 4 we explored the value of developing shared understandings through frequent and informal interactions with caregivers. Frequent and informal interactions can form a potent conduit enabling the caregivers to share their perspective and so feel included in the caregiving situation. As caregivers share stories in residential environments, so they share stories in community services. Many stories are biographical providing a window into their lives and relationships before caregiving. On an individual level, we listen to these stories and they form part of a shared history and shared understanding with the individual worker. As in residential care, it is vital that we apply these stories to the caregiving situation in community contexts to ensure caregivers are provided with support that meets their needs as well as the needs of the person living with dementia.

Partnership working

Therapeutic relationships where all perspectives are recognised and valued are central to partnerships with caregivers. To achieve partnership working, open and responsive communication enabling negotiation and compromise is required (Brown Wilson et al., 2009; Bramble et al., 2011). The responsibility of healthcare professionals such as nurses lies in the recognition of the expertise of the family caregiver as an ‘expert’ concerning the person with dementia (Nolan et al., 1996; Brown et al., 2001). This means that critical information is shared and its relevance recognised resulting in shared decision-making and

Table 8.1 Professional approaches to working with family caregivers

Approach	Types of interventions	Professional role
Facilitative	Planned, systematic and aims to facilitate the best outcome for carers and service users	Professionals acknowledge the expert knowledge of carers
Contributory	Interventions occur by chance rather than being planned	Professional actively works to complement the carer's role
Inhibitory	Carers perceive the benefits of the intervention as outweighing the costs	Lack of choice offered to caregiver
Obstructive	Professionals are seen as directly trying to block carer's efforts by failing to draw on their expertise	Professionals perceive carers to be obstructive or simply not in need of help

Source: based on Brown et al. (2001).

trusting relationships (Nolan et al., 2003; Davies, 2003; Brown Wilson and Davies, 2009). Support may be required to enable caregivers to develop competence and self-confidence initially but the increasing expertise of caregivers over time also needs to be recognised by healthcare professionals (Nolan et al., 1996). The approach we adopt in working with caregivers may support or restrict partnership working as identified in Table 8.1.

A fundamental purpose of partnership working is to develop facilitative interventions. To achieve this we need to recognise the caregiver's perspective of caregiving and what might be influencing this. The caregiver perspective also needs to form part of the assessment and care delivery process (Davies, 2003). Using the information we have covered within this chapter, develop a partnership working guide for your individual practice (Activity 8.6).

Activity 8.6 Critical Thinking

Develop a strategy for partnership working with the caregiver using the following headings:

Assessment:

- What are the issues from the perspective of the caregiver?
- What promotes the caregiver's wellbeing?
- What influences the stress experienced?

Planning:

- How is the caregiver's expertise valued and included?
- What are the caregiver's points of reference; what do they need increased/decreased?
- How is biography being shared and used?

(Continued)

(Continued)

Implementation:

- How does the care reflect the caregiver's perspective?
- Does it include:
    - Social support for the caregiver?
    - Education and skills training for the caregiver?
    - Positive events for both the person with dementia and the caregiver?

Evaluation:

- What are the outcomes defined by the caregiver?
- How are the caregiver's judgements included?

Conclusion

Relationship-based approaches to care require contribution from families and so we need to recognise the expertise of the family caregiver within dementia care. In the community, family caregivers provide care and support enabling the person with dementia to remain in the community. In doing this, caregivers become experts in caregiving and understanding the person with dementia. This means family caregivers are an absolute resource in enabling the professionals to deliver person-centred care. Although the person with dementia may be the focus of many services, relationship-centred care (Nolan et al., 2006b; Brown Wilson and Davies, 2009) recognises that there are times when the needs of caregivers need to be the primary focus. This chapter has examined the perspective of caregivers and the range of factors that affect their distress and their wellbeing, producing a strategy for partnership working.

Final reflections

In the previous chapter, we focused on the professional skills required in the delivery of relationship-based approaches to care. In this chapter, we have developed these skills to work collaboratively with caregivers. Although we may be tasked to provide services for the person with dementia, these interventions may be counterproductive if they do not take into account the caregiver perspective or their expertise. We have now developed a strategy for including the caregiver perspective as part of the assessment and care delivery process, which supports relationship-based approaches to care by taking into account all perspectives in the relationship.

Further reading

STAR-C

This website gives an overview of the community-based caregiver intervention developed by Linda Teri and colleagues: www.rosalynncarter.org/caregiver_intervention_database/dimentia/star-c_intervention/ (accessed 27/01/17).

Overview of REACH I and II studies

http://oafc.stanford.edu/projects/reach.html (accessed 27/01/17).

An overview of NYUCI

www.rosalynncarter.org/caregiver_intervention_database/dimentia/nyu_caregiver_counseling_and_support_intervention/ (accessed 27/01/17).

Social Care Institute for Excellence Dementia Gateway

A guide to working in partnership with caregivers. Available at: www.scie.org.uk/dementia/carers-of-people-with-dementia/ (accessed 27/01/17).

9

The role of technology in dementia care

Learning objectives

By the end of this chapter, the reader will be able to:

- Explore current debates about the ethics of technology in dementia care.
- Examine the use of technology in dementia care.
- Consider how technology may be used to promote relationship-based approaches to care.
- Develop a user involvement plan to engage the person with dementia and their families in the use of technology.

Introduction

Technology is ubiquitous in the twenty-first century with young adults who cannot remember life before the internet. Indeed, telling my students that I remember a time before Google places me in the same sphere as the older people I nursed in the 1980s as a young adult, who would tell me about their experiences in the first ever aeroplane and driving the very first car. As an even younger person, I remember my grandmother telling me about her life as a housewife before the labour saving technologies of refrigeration and washing machines. Technology or the concept of technology is not new; the scale, the speed and sophistication of technology, however, is markedly different in this century compared to the last. Marc Prensky (2001) speaks about 'Digital natives' as compared to 'Digital immigrants'. Those children born into the digital age (Digital natives) interact with the world and learn in a very different way from those of us described as 'Digital immigrants' who tend to learn in a step-by-step fashion (Prensky, 2001). This doesn't mean 'Digital immigrants' do not embrace technology but they will use technology differently (Prensky, 2001).

This is a critical point in understanding how technology may be embraced and accepted (or not) by older people with dementia.

Once a technology is developed, is intuitive to use and makes our lives easier, it soon becomes an integral part of our lives – such as the mobile phone. Wearable technology is now becoming the norm as many people use tracking devices, for example to monitor exercise and activity. Digitalisation and miniaturisation are also opening up whole new fields of development. 'Smart' technologies such as Artificial Intelligence (AI) are becoming increasingly commonplace where a machine is able to create new knowledge and so 'learn' by processing a series of algorithms much more quickly than a human brain. AI as an example has real potential for saving time in healthcare processes such as Emergency Triage. The rapid development of technology is creating new frontiers with which to support people with dementia. However, with development also comes potential dilemma particularly if we are considering how to implement relationship-based approaches to care.

Technologies are developed regularly but not all technologies will be adopted by those for whom they have been developed. Indeed those developing the technology may not fully understand the work processes, the environment, or the needs of the end user. When considering the development of technology in dementia care, involving the person with dementia, the family member and staff is vital to ensure the end product meets the needs of everyone who will be using the technology. There are a number of often overlapping reasons why technology is used in dementia care and in this chapter we will explore the overriding concern of safety and surveillance and whether this can equal independence for the person with dementia. The rights of people with dementia to take risks within their capabilities will also be explored in relation to the available technology.

Activity 9.1 Reflection

Who is technology serving?

Identify the technology currently in use in the organisation in which you practise and identify the benefits and concerns from each stakeholder's perspective:

	Technology	Benefits	Concerns
The organisation			
Staff providing care			
Family caregivers			
Person with dementia			

What issues are raised by using Assistive Technology in dementia care?

Technology is becoming a common feature of healthcare provision to monitor variables such as patient safety, activity patterns, sleeping characteristics, cognitive ability and changes in patient behaviour (Bharucha et al., 2009). Systems using Radio-Frequency IDentification (RFID) composed of tags, readers and servers, use radio waves to transfer data from a tag attached to people and are increasingly being used for real-time tracking of a person's movement (Bharucha et al., 2009). RFID tags are divided into two classes: active and passive, depending on how they are powered. Active tags have an integrated or replaceable battery which continuously powers the tag and its RF communication circuitry, thus allowing communication over a longer range and the incorporation of additional functionality such as memory and sensor devices. Passive tags have no internal power supply; the reader is responsible for powering and communicating with the tag. Passive tags are limited in their functionality but are smaller in size, cheaper and have a longer life span than active tags (Want, 2006). When used in dementia care, the passive RFID tags can be worn by the person with dementia (Hanser et al., 2008), embedded in clothing (Miura et al., 2009) or incorporated into jewellery (Nomura and Yamaji, 2008) and the readers inserted into floor mats or located on the walls of the rooms and corridors of interest. Camera surveillance may also be used, for example in remote monitoring to reduce falling, panicking and wandering, particularly at night (Schikhof and Mulder, 2008; Schikhof et al., 2010). The increasing use of remote monitoring in people's homes is now enabling access to healthcare that might not otherwise have been possible. This may include the use of everyday technologies such as televisions and phones to maintain contact with both health services and their social network.

In dementias where there is progressive neurological reduction, mobility may be one of the last functions to be lost. Continued mobility may be the vehicle by which people with dementia retain a key feature of their independence and thus their ability to make decisions that influence their wellbeing. Cognitive loss in dementia precipitates issues with recognition of familiar environments and wayfinding that are a major risk factor in residential admissions due to safety concerns, particularly when family caregivers feel unable to cope with this pattern of behaviour (van Hoof et al., 2007). The risk of a person with dementia becoming lost has given rise to the development of surveillance technologies to maintain safety and enable people with dementia to remain living in the community (Godwin, 2012; Zwijsen et al., 2012). Maintaining independence and improving quality of life for the person with dementia are suggested benefits of employing surveillance technology although few studies have been able to demonstrate such benefits (Niemeijer et al., 2010). The main concern regarding surveillance technologies in the literature is the autonomy of the person with dementia versus the duty of care that staff need to exercise to ensure safety (Niemeijer et al., 2010). This overriding concern for safety may result in staff using sensor technology as a restraint rather than enabling the person with dementia to move freely (Godwin, 2012; Zwijsen et al., 2012). Concerns have also been raised that Assistive Technology may reduce contact between staff members and the person with dementia which promotes positive relationships, with such technology possibly impeding the implementation of person-centred care (Savenstedt et al., 2006; Niemeijer et al., 2010; Zwijsen et al., 2012). Ethical issues are not well addressed within the literature (Niemeijer et al., 2010; Zwijsen et al., 2012) and older people themselves may potentially accept AT in an effort to avoid admission to a nursing home (Zwijsen et al., 2012). However, not all technology may prevent people with dementia from being admitted to residential care (Godwin, 2012) and concerns over safety continue to be a feature in the residential environment (Van Hoof et al., 2007).

Technology for surveillance and safety

A common focus of technology in residential environments for people living with dementia is the prevention of falls and subsequent injury. The concern about the risk of falls may result in enforced restrictions on the person with dementia with subsequent accelerated loss of function, so increasing disability (van Hoof et al., 2007).

Holmes et al. (2007) evaluated an integrated RFID system that comprised a bed exit sensor positioned under each resident's bed sheet in conjunction with bathroom and bedroom exit monitors that alerted caregivers via a silent pager when a high-risk resident exited his or her bed, bedroom or bathroom. Only one outcome (improved mood related to sleep quality) was found to be improved with no change being found in falls, behaviour or staff outcomes. This may be due to concerns staff had in trusting the technology, which resulted in them continuing to check on people rather than wait until the technology alerted them (Holmes et al., 2007). Also, staff considered a limitation of Assistive Technology was its inability to prevent falls or adverse events and that it did not always guarantee someone receiving timely assistance due to multiple alarms going off simultaneously (Zwijsen et al., 2012). Engstrom et al. (2009) interviewed staff to identify their perception of the implementation of similar technology (passage alarms, sensor activated night time illumination, and fall detectors). Staff identified how the system enabled people with dementia to make decisions about their location without staff being concerned about the person with dementia's safety. This was echoed in a study that considered how access technology influenced the wellbeing of the person with dementia where it was suggested that access control technology promoted autonomy of movement for the person with dementia as well as providing a sense of security for staff (Margot-Cattin and Nygard, 2006). This technology involved a RFID card on the person with dementia that opened the door to their room but then locked the doors to the external environment. Staff considered that this system supported the capability of the person with dementia in their integration into the environment (Margot-Cattin and Nygard, 2006).

Part of the concerns with safety in residential environments is ensuring people with dementia remain in the care environment. Technology is commonly used to alert staff when a person begins to leave a care environment. Aud (2004) conducted a retrospective review of 62 elopement incidents using case records, where 32% of cases resulted in injury to the resident. The technology included alarms on doorways that alerted staff when the door was opened, or when residents wearing a sensor approached or exited through a door. Subsequently the study identified key areas of concern in how staff used this technology; particularly regarding the active ignoring of alarms or difficulty in hearing them (Aud, 2004). In an ethnographic study, Wigg (2010) considered the impact of locked doors compared with motion sensors which detected when a person had left the premises, alerting staff to join them and guide them back to the home. In Wigg's (2010) study, locked doors created a sense of frustration with people with dementia trying the door or milling around looking for ways to exit the premises. This study suggested that motion detection promoted a person's autonomy in where they chose to walk with staff being alerted if there was the risk of harm. Chen et al. (2007) used video to detect behaviour around doorways that may lead to elopement and this prompted alerts to staff. RFID tags are also used to detect elopement and their use in a day care centre in Taiwan provided the people with dementia with more freedom to move around the building without staff becoming anxious (Lin et al., 2008). These studies demonstrate the potential for AT to facilitate interaction with the physical environment by removing potential barriers to activity due to locked doors (Margot-Cattin and Nygard, 2006; Chen et al., 2007; Lin et al., 2008; Engstrom et al., 2009; Wigg, 2010) resulting in less agitation (Wigg, 2010). Enabling people with dementia to choose where they go within an environment was considered to facilitate independence (Engstrom et al., 2009; Wigg, 2010) thus providing residents with feelings of security and achievement (Margot-Cattin and Nygard, 2006). Residential care staff also described how people with dementia who were walking to different areas within the home appeared happier with this freedom (Margot-Cattin and Nygard, 2006; Engstrom et al., 2009).

Motion patterns using RFID tags (sewn into the resident's collar) with readers (Greiner et al., 2007) demonstrated to staff that the patterns of movement of people with dementia were purposeful, rather than aimless wandering. This was achieved by creating a graphic display of residents' movement pattern that was then sent to a computer at the nurses' station. The study concluded that patterns of movement can be understood in respect to a person's previous behaviours. Similarly, a longitudinal study of resident data (30 months) using a system of under flooring pressure sensors and tags in residents' slippers (Miura et al., 2009) suggested that mobility patterns may be linked to seasonal variations or changes in condition (Fujinami et al., 2011). Whilst technology provides us with this critical information, graphic displays are meaningless unless something is done with the information provided by the technology that improves the quality of life for the person with dementia. A group of researchers in Austria used a technological system to improve the quality of life for people living in a dementia unit. Using a combination of tags, accelerometers and microphones, information was gathered on social interaction, aggressive behaviour, the quality of sleep and where residents liked to spend their day (Hanser et al., 2008; Grünerbl et al., 2011). This information was used to identify motion patterns that represented positive, negative and neutral states of the person with dementia when compared with the medical notes. Grünerbl et al. (2011) suggest that this system may enable people with dementia to live their lives comfortably in small group homes without constant staff interaction, thus improving quality of life.

Schikhof and Mulder (2008) used Value Sensitive Design and a human-centred approach to design a technological solution that would meet the needs of all stakeholders in a dementia care unit. A central focus of this study was the mapping of values for all stakeholders and an iterative process of returning to stakeholders as the technology was developed and piloted to ensure that everyone's needs were being met in the final system. Video camera and infra-red technology were installed in resident bedrooms for use solely at night time, which was considered acceptable by both staff and family members. Following the implementation of this technology, staff and managers reported that the video camera technology provided more freedom by enabling the people with dementia to take acceptable risks (Schikhof et al., 2010).

Video cameras were also used to improve the quality of life for people with dementia in group homes in Japan by supporting staff in understanding the person with dementia (Takatsuka and Fujinami, 2005; Sugihara et al., 2008). Caregivers described improved decision-making and communication with the person with dementia, which changed the working patterns of staff, enabling the person with dementia to live more independently (Sugihara et al., 2008, Sugihara and Fujinami, 2011).

Does surveillance + safety = independence for the person with dementia?

The discussion in the previous section suggests that technology may facilitate the promotion of wellbeing for people with dementia in residential care environments by reducing barriers within the environment that impact on a person's functioning (Schneidert et al., 2003). There is some evidence for enhanced participation of people with dementia in the social context using surveillance technologies with two studies that demonstrated an enhanced capacity for the person with dementia to make choices as to where they wish to spend their time and who they wish to interact with (Hanser et al., 2008; Grünerbl et al., 2011). There was also some evidence that enabling staff to recognise problems remotely provides the person with dementia with greater freedom in their daily living (Grünerbl et al., 2008; Sugihara and Fujinami, 2011). However, in order to promote this level of independence using AT, privacy was often infringed through the use of video technologies (Bharucha et al., 2009). Privacy and autonomy are regular concerns in the AT literature with both family caregivers and staff often resistive to using video technology (Zwijsen et al., 2011).

Activity 9.2 Critical Thinking

Identify a person with dementia from your practice:

- What type of technology is being used to enhance their care?
- What additional technology might be used to increase their independence?
- What are the potential benefits and concerns that might emerge?

Type of technology	Purpose	Potential benefits	Potential concerns

Now consider:

- How would you measure the potential benefits?
- How would you monitor the potential concerns?

Technology to promote independence in the community

Technology embedded into a person's living environment that enables the interaction between technology and healthcare professionals is becoming widely accepted as a mechanism for improving health outcomes in Chronic Disease Management (Department of Health, 2011). For example, the Whole Systems Demonstrator (WSD) project in the UK demonstrated that using a range of embedded technology via tele-health substantially reduces mortality and hospital admissions for people living with chronic conditions (Department of Health, 2011). The term often used for these systems is Ambient Assisted Living (AAL) which refers to an ecosystem of sensors, computers, wireless networks, software applications and actuator networks (WSANs) which are interconnected to exchange data, which is then sent via a gateway to provide healthcare services. AAL is an integrated system of systems (Memon et al., 2014). AAL systems should be developed with the end user having a focus on usability and dependability. In particular, technological solutions should be non-invasive, embedded into the environment and adaptive to the end user's needs (Cavallo et al., 2015). In a review of the AAL literature, Memon et al. (2014) found that few studies fully explored the end-user experience and there was a dearth of participatory approaches to the development process. Pol et al. (2016) report that community dwelling seniors use sensor technology in their homes to feel a sense of safety and to continue living independently. The older people in this sample felt that capturing movement did not infringe their privacy and enabled the healthcare professional to provide advice on how to keep active (Pol et al., 2016).

Cavallo et al. (2015) suggest there needs to be a user-centred design approach including a multidisciplinary team involving the older person. We saw this approach earlier in the design of a system for a residential dementia unit (Schikhof and Mulder, 2008). Working with people living with dementia in the community, Roger Orpwood and colleagues at the Bath Institute of Medical Engineering use a participatory design approach that enables the person with dementia to lead the research process by identifying the issues they find challenging and for which a technological solution might be found (Orpwood et al., 2010). A participatory approach involving people living with dementia needs to be an integral feature of developing relevant and usable systems that will have meaning for people living with dementia and their caregivers. Similarly, Evans et al. (2011) evaluated a range of sensors that was designed to improve the independence and quality of life for a person with dementia. A system of automatic lighting, motion sensors and voice reminders alerted staff when there was a problem, enabling the person with dementia to live more independently. Cavallo et al. (2015) developed a system for people living with dementia that included iterative development with extensive involvement of professional and family caregivers in the design and piloting phases to ensure the system could be integrated into the life of the person with dementia as well as the services being delivered. The purpose of this project was to integrate technology in such a way as to maintain and enhance functional health, security, safety, and quality of life for people living with dementia. This was achieved using a range of wearable devices alongside smart environments that continuously monitor the person's activities and physical status, adapting the environment and providing proactive supportive measures (Cavallo et al., 2015). Whilst the level of independence achieved is high in this project, the loss of privacy is also high. Herein lies the dilemma as to whether the infringement on privacy will lead to a loss of autonomy or the ability of the person with dementia to make their own decisions.

In a number of studies that have explored caregiver perceptions of technology, each study reports that family caregivers are more likely to suggest the infringement of the person with dementia's privacy and autonomy when compared to issues of safety (Robinson et al., 2007; Olsson et al., 2012; Mao et al., 2015). This is because family caregivers find it immensely challenging to maintain a sense of safety and security in their daily lives when faced with the unpredictability of how dementia influences the behaviour of the person they are caring for (Robinson et al., 2007; Olsson et al., 2012). Professional caregivers tend to give more weight to autonomy over security suggesting a person-centred approach should be adopted before implementing tracking devices (Robinson et al., 2007). People with dementia refer to the value of being able to go out of doors independently but suggest they find mobile devices confusing and difficult to use (Robinson et al., 2007). The use of GPS technology remains a common debate when supporting people with dementia (Landau et al., 2010; Magnusson et al., 2014). Whilst a predominant benefit of GPS technology is the family caregivers' peace of mind, professional caregivers' views change according to the locus of responsibility with patient safety overshadowing autonomy when the professional caregiver has primary responsibility for the person with dementia (Landau et al., 2010). A Swedish Demonstration Project for people living with dementia across twelve municipalities reveals mixed reports between the professional and family caregivers and the person with dementia using GPS technology (Magnusson et al., 2014). Lennart Magnusson and colleagues (2014) developed an Extended Safety and Support (ESS) system using a participatory approach involving people with dementia, family caregivers and the staff supporting them. The ESS system was not considered to be an intrusion of privacy for the majority of people with dementia involved in the study. Although the amount of times the person with dementia accessed the outdoors decreased over the length of the study, possibly due to disease progression, family caregivers reported the person with dementia was able to be more independent when they did engage in outdoor activities (Magnusson et al., 2014). Professional caregivers believed the ESS system enabled the person with dementia to remain in their home for longer. However, professional caregivers also had greater concerns for privacy issues when compared to the person with dementia or their family caregiver, which may impact on whether AT is recommended or supported by professional caregivers. The discrepancy between the views of professional and family caregivers is well documented in the literature (Robinson et al., 2007). The ESS study (Magnusson et al., 2014) suggests the value of undertaking individual and person-centred assessments to ensure the views of the person with dementia as well as the family caregiver are taken into account when making decisions about the use of AT. The following activity supports you in thinking about the potential technology may have to promote relationship-based approaches to care.

Activity 9.3 Critical Thinking

Use of technology to enhance the opportunity for person-centred practice

Consider how technology might be used to facilitate the following aspects of person-centred care:

- Getting to know the person – using the information from informal care interactions to support the ongoing development of care planning.
- Attention to significant details – with attention to the biography of the person.
- Anticipating needs – with attention to the social environment.

How might the person with dementia and their family contribute to this process using technology?

Consider how technology might be used to facilitate relationship-centred care:

- How might the information from person-centred care be shared across the team and between shifts to develop shared understandings?
- How might information be shared informally and frequently using technology to enable responsive care:

  - between staff?
  - including families?
  - including the person with dementia?

- How might the contribution of the person with dementia and families to the community be facilitated using technology?

Return to Activity 9.2 – consider the types of technology in that list and compare their function to what is needed in the current list. Are there other technologies that need to be explored?

The next section of this chapter will explore how AAL environments have been developed to improve health outcomes in Assisted Living (AL) environments. AL environments enable older people to live independently within individual units providing access to shared social spaces and healthcare. In the US, the University of Missouri have created 'Tiger Place', an AL environment that provides state-of-the-science care alongside the opportunity for residents to be involved in cutting-edge research.

Practice scenario 9.1

Tiger Place is an Assisted Living environment jointly managed by a private healthcare provider and the University of Missouri. The aim of Tiger Place is to promote the health and independence of older people for as long as possible. The objective is to enable older people to 'Age in Place'. To fully provide the best research-informed practice, Tiger Place also provides a research environment where technology and care interventions can be developed and evaluated whilst ensuring the residents have access to cutting-edge care. In this context, research is undertaken in collaboration with residents and only residents who provide informed consent are involved in the research. Over the past 10 years, within Tiger Place, there has been the development and implementation of a range of sensor technology that passively and unobtrusively collects information about patterns of movement, activity and sleeping patterns through motion sensors, bed sensors and Microsoft Kinect. Video sensors only extract silhouettes or other graphical representation to maintain privacy. This information is analysed via a behaviour reasoning component that can generate alerts. Information is sent to a database through a wireless internet connection with a secure web-based interface available for viewing by residents, families and healthcare professionals. This system is used in conjunction with a system of electronic health records and Registered Nurse Care co-ordination to improve health outcomes of the residents. All residents receive a comprehensive health assessment on admission and thereafter every six months from a Registered Nurse who is available 24 hours a day/7 days per week. In addition residents have access to health promotion activities and a social worker to support life transitions.

Source: based on Rantz et al. (2005).

Residents in Tiger Place were invited to focus groups to identify their preferences for the use of AT and opted not to wear devices but accepted installed unobtrusive devices. Cameras were also considered acceptable as long as they only captured the silhouette of the person. Data are collected from an apartment and displayed in a map of activity, the density of which can be captured across a 24-hour period. In this way, the activity of a person can be compared over time with any changes being sent automatically as an alert to the Registered Nurse Care Coordinator (Rantz et al., 2005, 2013a 2015b; Popescu and Mahnot, 2012).

The sensor technology at Tiger Place has been used to detect subtle changes in older people that might not be immediately apparent (Rantz et al., 2011) alerting caregivers earlier in the trajectory of illness thus enabling them to provide timely treatment, preventing potential decline in mobility and independence (Alexander et al., 2011; Rantz et al., 2012, 2015b). A series of case studies from Tiger Place demonstrate how sensor technology can collate patterns of activity, documenting changes in behavioural patterns indicating urinary tract infections (Rantz et al., 2011) and mental health, including dementia (Galambos et al., 2013) with subsequent work in detecting risk of falls (Rantz et al., 2015a).

As changes in a person's cognitive status may present in diverse ways, the key aspect of this system is to be able to identify a person's usual pattern before the onset of decline (Rantz et al., 2015b). Retrospective data for residents with a diagnosis of dementia demonstrated a pattern of changing activity both within the apartment and in taking opportunities to leave their apartment (Galambos et al., 2013). Once additional care was implemented, the data can then be analysed to chart improvement in the person with dementia's activity patterns, demonstrating the effectiveness of the treatment. Density maps provide a visual display that could act as prompts for healthcare professionals to undertake mental health assessment and implement treatment earlier in the trajectory of illness (Galambos et al., 2013).

Companion technology is another emerging field where the system adapts to the user's needs thus creating a smart human–technology interaction (Biundo et al., 2016). Companion systems may focus on conversational interaction or provide support for activities of daily living (Bemelmans et al., 2012). Kerssens et al. (2015) developed an in-house system to deliver personalised support in the management of Neuropsychiatric symptoms (NPS) within the home environment. The 'Companion' is a touch screen computer based on reminiscence of a person's life story, customised to activities and memories that provide pleasure. The purpose was for the person with dementia to use this independently and so provide meaningful activity. Caregivers and the people with dementia using this technology were overwhelmingly positive although it did not increase the person with dementia's independence from the caregiver's perspective (Kerssens et al., 2015).

Other types of companion technology include animal robots. Libin and Cohen-Mansfield (2004) provided a group of people living with dementia in nursing homes with either a toy plush cat or a robotic cat and found that both reduced agitation and increased pleasure when the person with dementia interacted with either cat. A well known companion robot in dementia care is the Paro seal (Wada et al., 2007, 2008). Paro is designed as a baby harp seal to avoid preconceptions that may come with other animals and is designed with a behaviour generation system. This means that the seal can respond to interactions via inbuilt sensors (sight, auditory, balance and tactile) (Wada et al., 2008). Paro was given to a day centre where people with dementia engaged regularly with the seal. Urine tests suggested the people with dementia were less stressed and the staff also reported less stress using a burnout scale (Wada et al., 2004). Although no structured tests were undertaken, Paro's use in one institution for five years suggested residents interacted regularly with Paro, reporting it made them feel happier (Wada et al., 2009). There have been few structured studies in assessing the effectiveness of Paro, with the majority being observational studies focusing on increased social interaction between residents (Kidd et al., 2006; Wada et al., 2007). Professor Wendy Moyle undertook a pilot randomised controlled trial (RCT) in Australia in 2013, comparing the effects of Paro to a structured reading group (Moyle et al., 2013a). The group receiving Paro improved in their quality of life and pleasure scores and there is a larger trial underway (Moyle et al., 2015).

A recurrent theme throughout this chapter has been user-centred design, involving the person with dementia and their caregivers at all points in the design process, from conception through to user interface to ensure the technology meets the needs of those for whom it is intended (Schikhof and Mulder, 2008; Bharucha et al., 2009). User-centred design also enables people with dementia to have a voice in what matters to them (Magnusson et al., 2014). Returning to our lens of Complex Adaptive Systems, utilising multidisciplinary groups including the end user provides for greater cognitive diversity, resulting in novel and creative solutions ensuring the end product remains usable and feasible (Bangar et al., 2015; Cavallo et al., 2015).

Practice scenario 9.2

Developing technology using partnerships

This project started with a watermelon and a can of Coke to demonstrate the potential for a collection of polymer optic fibres to capture the weight of objects and transfer these into images using tomographic imaging principles.

I was involved in convening a multi-professional group including people with dementia, family caregivers, care managers, researchers and health professionals to identify the potential use for this technology in dementia care. The potential for this technology to record changes in pressure distribution of foot balance, step sequence and position in real time suggested it could be developed into a 'SMART' carpet, which the engineers then built with input from health professionals and a person with dementia who was an engineer. Data were then collected to identify how the system communicates changes in gait pattern leading to a fall.

(Continued)

(Continued)

These findings were presented to focus groups comprised of people with dementia, family caregivers and professionals from the NHS and private care sector. The objective of these focus groups was to evaluate the utility of this system for clinical practice including the acceptability of this technology for people with dementia and family caregivers.

People with dementia, family caregivers and staff identify the relevance of technology that can alert them prior to an incident such as a fall occurring. Embedded optical fibres in a mat or underlay can be used to non-intrusively collect data over time without infringement on privacy. Clinical staff can use a sequence of images that identify changes in walking patterns to identify risk factors that may precipitate a fall. However, further development of predictive capacity would be needed for utility in the clinical environment. Involving people with dementia, family caregivers and clinical staff in the development of technology at an early stage, significantly enhances the likelihood of such developed technology meeting the needs of the end users in healthcare.

Activity 9.4

Using technology with people living with dementia

Develop a plan that enables the perspective of the person with dementia and the family caregiver to be included in the decision-making process for use of technology:

1. What is the purpose of using the technology?
2. What are the ethical implications of using this technology? How might these be addressed?
3. What are the risks in not using the technology being considered?
4. How did the person with dementia interact with technology before they were diagnosed with dementia?
5. Has the technology been discussed with the person with dementia and their family caregivers?
6. Will the technology enhance the person with dementia's life? If so, how?

Conclusion

Assistive technology is becoming increasingly sophisticated as we move through the twenty-first century. Older people and those living with dementia may be digital immigrants but this does not mean they do not engage with technology. Technology has the potential to promote independence but in doing this it might also infringe the privacy and autonomy of the person with dementia. Whilst surveillance technologies can be used to collect a range of data to improve health outcomes, there remain issues around privacy and autonomy. Whilst different stakeholders will view the balance of risk differently it is vital that all perspectives are included when making the decision whether to use technology.

Final reflections

Technology is a ubiquitous feature of modern living. With advances in technology come ethical and moral debates about the inclusion of the person with dementia in being able to make decisions that affect their right to autonomy within their decision-making capacity. We have seen in this chapter the potential for technology to contribute to relationship-based approaches to care by enabling the transfer of information for responsive care decisions to be made. Equally, there is a role for technology in promoting the contribution of the person with dementia and their family caregivers by capturing the stories they share. The potential for technology to improve health outcomes is compelling for healthcare professionals, yet this must never overshadow the risks to privacy and autonomy. The Registered Nurse is in a unique position in this debate to enable the involvement of the person with dementia in the decision-making process. The following chapter will take you through how this might be achieved.

Further reading

Assistive technology for people with dementia

This website contains a range of information including a directory of services, access to research and development, as well as information on the ethical use of technology and how to obtain Assistive Technology. Available at: www.atdementia.org.uk (accessed 27/01/17).

Centre for Eldercare and Rehabilitation Technology, University of Missouri

An interdisciplinary group of faculty, staff and students who are focused on investigating, developing and evaluating technology to serve the needs of older adults and others with physical and cognitive challenges. Research results are disseminated and effective technologies are translated to commercialisation to serve those in need. New healthcare technologies, driven by actual clinical needs, are developed and evaluated in real world settings. Available at: www.eldertech.missouri.edu/ (accessed 27/01/17).

Bath Institute of Medical Engineering (BIME)

BIME is a design and development charity working alongside various partners to promote and establish the potential of using new technology in the field of dementia care. Available at: www.bath.ac.uk/health/about/partner-organisations/designability/ (accessed 27/01/17).

Paro seal

This website explains the design of Paro with access to a range of research papers. Available at: www.parorobots.com/ (accessed 27/01/17).

Companion robots

Professor Wendy Moyle from Griffith University, Australia speaks about her work with robot therapy and people with dementia. The video also demonstrates the different robots involved in the programme of research. Available at: www.youtube.com/watch?v=UklgDdcf02Q (accessed 27/01/17).

10

Leading and managing change in dementia care

Learning objectives

By the end of this chapter, the reader will be able to:

- Examine how leadership for change might be used to promote relationship-centred care.
- Apply the principles of culture change and what this means for managing change in practice.
- Explore the role of quality improvement cycles in promoting relationship-based dementia care.
- Develop a quality improvement cycle that promotes a relationship-based approach to dementia care.

Introduction

Throughout this book we have considered organisations as Complex Adaptive Systems (CAS) and explored how each level (*micro–meso–macro*) of the organisation facilitates relationship-based approaches to dementia care. We began this book by exploring the value of flexibility and how staff can be supported to move along a continuum between individualised, person-centred and relationship-centred care. A key assumption behind the concept of this continuum is enabling staff to work flexibly, ensuring that leadership at each level of the organisation is promoting relationship-based care. The tendency in dementia care environments is to adopt a hierarchical bureaucratic model that meets rules and regulations thus creating a focus on the task. We saw that adopting the principles of CAS for dementia care organisations facilitates open communication, enabling the development of responsive relationships between staff who are encouraged to self-organise. Facilitating decision-making to include all levels of staff, people with dementia and families enables everyone to actively make a contribution and so develop personal, responsive and reciprocal relationships (Brown Wilson et al., 2009). The contribution from people with dementia and their families includes biographical stories that support staff in implementing person-centred and relationship-centred care. Using the principles of CAS introduces staff to new ways of working together in implementing relationship-based approaches to care.

Dementia care is becoming a highly politicised business endeavour with businesses espousing the language of person-centred care. Although some organisations may have person-centred philosophies, this is not always reflected in direct care with staff in some of the studies we have reviewed citing lack of management support as a key barrier (Moyle et al., 2013b). We have also reviewed strategies integral to the management and leadership of teams to ensure staff are supported in the implementation of relationship-based approaches to care. Informal, frequent communication between staff and managers allowed problem solving that encouraged staff to identify solutions and so adapt their working to meet the changing needs of people with dementia and their families. Leading by example with the role modelling of person-centred care facilitated the team in providing a consistent approach that promoted relationship-based approaches to care.

Decisions at each level of the organisation may support or hinder the ability of staff to work flexibly, communicate openly and so create new ways of working through self-organisation. In this chapter, we will connect the language of relationships and self-organisation with that of Quality Improvement (QI). We will explore how QI methodology may be used at different levels of the organisation to facilitate culture change and so promote relationship-based dementia care. Using the principles of organisations as CAS, we will develop Quality Improvement Cycles for each level of the organisation to facilitate relationship-based approaches to care across the organisation. QI is a practice imperative and nurses are in a strong position to use QI to lead and manage change thus promoting improved outcomes for people living with dementia and their families. The focus in this book has been how to implement relationship-based approaches to care from an organisational perspective. The end point is to influence improved outcomes in dementia care for the person with dementia, their families and staff. This may necessitate change and that warrants leadership, so we will now explore how the two are connected.

Leadership for change

Leadership and management are often used synonymously but represent different concepts. Both leadership and management are critical for complex organisations to perform well in constantly changing markets. Care organisations operate in an increasingly competitive and challenging marketplace. This requires effective management to ensure quality processes are working well alongside leadership that enables organisations to take advantage of opportunities to improve (Kotter International, 2012). Managers might not always consider that leadership is part of their job whereas staff prefer clear leadership from their manager (Sellgren et al., 2008).

Leaders create vision and strategy, motivating people to action by communicating and setting direction so that people behave in different ways for improved outcomes.

Managers focus on the organisation of what needs to be done, thus resulting in improved outcomes. So whilst the end result of improved outcomes is similar, the way a manager might arrive at that outcome could be very different to a leader. I like to think that the manager is concentrating on 'what' needs to be done whereas the leader is focusing on 'how' it can be achieved. In this context, it is distinctly possible for one person to be performing the two roles. There are many theories of leadership but we have implicitly been discussing leadership styles throughout this book. Style theory suggests that leadership is not about having traits or being 'born to lead' but is about behaviours. This means that differing leadership styles may be required for different situations and that leaders can then adopt differing ways of working. There are two key sets of behaviours that represent leadership styles: task-focused and relationship-focused. Leadership style is considered more effective when leaders adopt different styles according to the situation (Goleman, 2000) and this variation in style will maintain a balance between the focus on the task and the focus on relationships (Hersey et al., 2001). Hersey et al. (2001) present a model of situated leadership (Figure 10.1) which identifies that task behaviours, such as the amount of direction required, and relationship behaviours, such as the amount of support given, need to be balanced alongside the confidence and competence of the follower to do the job (Hersey et al., 2001). This inherent flexibility of leadership complements the concept that relationship-based approaches to care can operate along a continuum with the approach to care adjusting according to the situation (refer back to Figure 2.5). This means that leaders will also require a flexible pattern of leadership behaviour if they are supporting staff in moving along the continuum when implementing person-centred or relationship-centred care.

Throughout this book, we have considered organisations as being Complex Adaptive Systems (CAS). Snowden and Boone (2007) suggest that the role of the leader in a complex environment is to create an environment that allows patterns to emerge by increasing levels of interaction and communication. In Chapter 4 we examined how the increased informal interactions between staff, managers and families promoted shared understandings, subsequently leading to responsive patterns of working. As we begin to think about Quality Improvement, we should view this as an important feature of CAS and as such, it needs to be built into the change management process. There is always a risk that leaders fall back to a more task-focused, command and respond mentality (Snowden and Boone, 2007), which might be equated with 'Leading from the front' when we are thinking of dementia care (Brown Wilson, 2009). There may be times when a task focus is needed such as when there are inexperienced staff who lack confidence. On these occasions it may be appropriate to be more directive in how to approach specific care tasks. However if we are working within an organisation that is implementing relationship-based approaches, then this should result in an individualised approach to care, rather than a task focus. 'Leading by example' (Brown Wilson, 2009) was discussed in Chapter 5 as an effective mode of leadership to implement relationship-based approaches to care. Leading by example might be described as a coaching style of leadership which aims to support staff in achieving their potential and take responsibility for their practice (Goleman, 2000; Connor and Pakora, 2007). However, there may exist organisational structures that obstruct practices such as

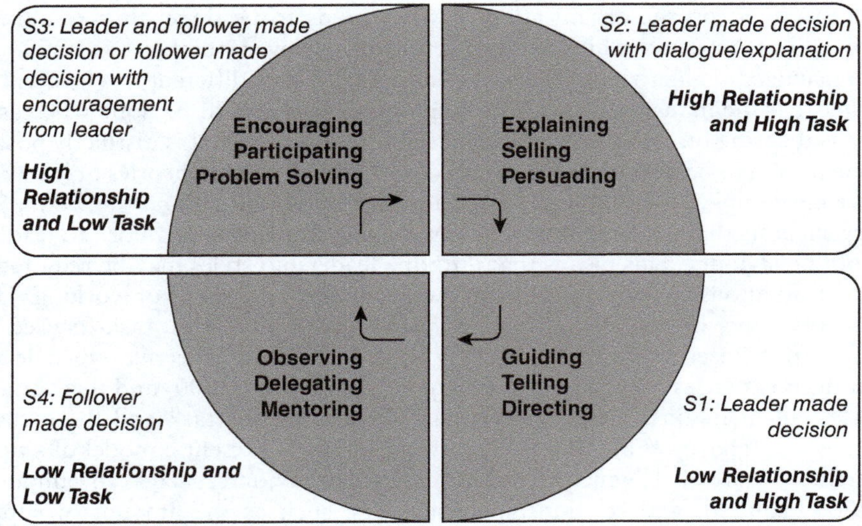

Figure 10.1 Model of situated leadership, Hersey et al. (2001)

open and responsive communication or flexible working practices and we will explore how we might identify and address these potential obstacles as we progress through this chapter. Team coaching is one strategy that could be adopted to enable teams to realign themselves with the articulated vision of relationship-based approaches to care whereby managers are available to individually coach staff as required (Connor and Pakora, 2007). Risk taking by trying new ways of working also needs to be encouraged, enabling staff to work collaboratively and flexibly so patterns can emerge. New ways of working require appropriate support by managers, alongside regular team meetings that promote interaction and enable cognitive diversity in developing solutions (Snowden and Boone, 2007). Not all managers readily buy into a change process and this may become evident through their failure to remove organisational barriers thus blocking change (Kotter, 2007). Such blocking behaviour needs to be addressed by honest and open dialogue to ensure the teams are supported in realising the solutions they have identified (Kotter, 2007; Kotter and Whitehead, 2010).

As with the continuum of care, where we may move from individualised to person-centred and on to relationship-centred care, so too can leadership progress from a task focus to a relational focus as staff develop both competence and confidence (Hersey et al., 2001). The key for leadership in dementia care is for leaders to be able to accurately assess what style of leadership is needed at what point. When reviewing nursing styles of leadership, Brady Germain and Cummings (2010) found that relationally-focused leadership led to positive outcomes for staff and the nursing work environment, when compared to a task-focused leadership style. Relationship-oriented leadership in nursing homes in the US also demonstrated improved resident outcomes (Anderson and McDaniel, 1998). Further to this, Brady Germain and Cummings (2010) also found that relational leadership styles increased nurses' research utilisation thus promoting evidence-based practice. Overall, change-oriented leadership appears to result in a better organisational culture. In the next section of this chapter, we will explore the role of culture change and how this might facilitate an organisational approach to relationship-based dementia care.

Culture change

Internationally, the culture change movement is gathering pace and within the US alone, over 85% of residential aged care facilities are involved in some form of culture change (Miller et al., 2014b). Culture change is an intentional choice by an organisation to become less institutional and more resident directed, empowering staff in making decisions about the care they deliver (Miller et al., 2014a). In the UK, a number of programmes have been initiated to improve quality of care and quality of life in long-term care environments:

- My Home Life network works with care homes to implement an evidence-based framework for improved quality of care and quality of life (Owen, 2006);
- The Pearl (Positively Enriching and Enhancing Resident's Lives) Programme has also been implemented across a large-scale provider (Baker, 2009);
- The Butterfly Programme provides an organisational approach to implementing activity within a person-centred framework of care (Sheard, 2014).

Each of the above models promotes the refocus of the organisation on the person receiving care using strategies to improve self-identity, develop opportunities for meaningful activity and focus on person-centred or relationship-centred care principles. Essentially any organisation can embark on culture change, but for those that wish to be endorsed as following a particular model of care, there is a more stringent process, a subscription fee and subsequent support in the implementation phase. Culture change including the use of subscription-based models is well established within the US Long-Term Care sector. However, Petriwskyj et al. (2016b) found that there were often differences in how the same model of culture change was implemented with limited evidence for improved resident and family or staff outcomes (Petriwskyj et al., 2016a).

For organisations to embark on culture change there are six key principles that need to be incorporated into practice to create a more resident-centred environment including: having residents directing activities; providing a homelike atmosphere; close relationships between staff, residents and families; collaborative decision-making; staff empowerment and quality improvement (Koren, 2010). In a large US-based survey, Miller et al. (2014a) asked Directors of Nursing Homes to assess the level of culture change the home was embarking on and then compared these findings to the quality indicators reviewed by the regulatory authority. Miller et al. (2014a) found that higher levels of implementation of culture change were positively associated with improved quality processes and outcomes. Further findings suggest that there were fewer deficiencies found by regulatory bodies, demonstrating how organisations that are actively implementing a high level of culture change can improve their quality indicators (Miller et al., 2014a). This is a powerful lever for leading and managing change in organisations. In the following activity, we will explore the different practices we have seen that might lend themselves to culture change.

Activity 10.1 Reflection

Complete the following table:

Principles of a culture change approach	**Examples from the literature**	**Provide an example of observed practice in an organisation in which you have practised**
Resident directed care	Activities should where possible be directed by the residents	
Home-like atmosphere	Small household units would be ideal, with opportunities for preparation of meals and/ or snacks on the unit	
Close relationships	Relationships between residents, staff, families and community should be fostered and encouraged through activities such as regular staff assignments	
Staff empowerment	Teamwork should be encouraged in responding to residents' needs alongside regular staff training	
Collaborative decision-making	Participatory management systems should be encouraged with a flattening of the hierarchical nature of the organisation	
Systematic quality improvement	Measurable outcomes should be identified and used as ways of ensuring ongoing improvement	

Source: based on Koren (2010).

Decisions to belong to culture change groups are invariably made by senior management and present with a range of changes that involve staff such as staff scheduling, the wearing of uniforms and providing staff education (Banaszak-Holl et al., 2013). Therefore to enable such principles to be enacted, it would be necessary to have the support of management and for these principles to be reflected in the organisation's espoused vision, mission and policies. Therefore if we wish to promote change, as practitioners, we need to use the language of policies to create opportunities for change and QI provides us with a mechanism to achieve this. Many of the studies we have reviewed have struggled to consistently demonstrate measurable clinical outcomes for the person with dementia. However, care interactions and relationships do improve (Moyle et al., 2013b; Chenoweth et al., 2014; Killett et al., 2016) and case studies illustrate the individual benefits to people living with dementia and staff when adopting person-centred care (see Brooker and Latham, 2015). The premise throughout this book is that if we employ strategies at each level of the organisation then we are more likely to achieve relationship-based approaches to care. The final stage in this process is to consider how we might use QI methodology to influence change at each level of the organisation.

Quality improvement

Considering the *macro* level of an organisation, we have explored how the language of relationship-centred approaches to care could be reflected in policies. We have rejected the metaphor of organisations as machines in favour of the lens of Complex Adaptive Systems to enable staff to self-organise thus providing personal and responsive care. This is different to the language of change management in healthcare, which tends to focus on flow and process in a similar vein to the manufacturing industry following the machine metaphor, with the underpinning assumption that all processes occur in a linear fashion and that the end result can be predicted (Ben-Tovim et al., 2008). The continued use of the machine metaphor may be due to the focus all organisations have on delivering their primary task, which may override any desire for innovation. This may be explained to some extent by the regulatory demands made on health care and the importance places on such reviews by external bodies. Regulation is important to ensure that minimum standards are maintained in dementia care, but should not be used as an excuse not to improve or change the service. Indeed the regulatory authority could be considered an external force that might prompt the organisation to co-evolve as a Complex Adaptive System, using the feedback from the regulatory report.

Quality standards tend to be translated into 'Key Performance Indicators' or 'KPIs' which are the quality measurements used to ensure the organisation meets regulatory requirements. These may vary between organisations depending on their overarching philosophy and whether the company holds charitable status, is 'for profit' or 'not for profit', or located in either the government or non-statutory sectors. In the case of dementia care, there exist external regulatory frameworks under which the business operates that will influence these KPIs. The regulatory framework may differ depending on the organisation in which you practise. Larger organisations may also manage these KPIs differently such as by giving individual working units specific KPIs by which their performance is measured. It is imperative that the focus on Quality Improvement is integrated into the relationship-based approaches to care or we run the risk of KPIs pulling us back to a task focus. Use the next activity to align the quality standards from your organisation to the six given areas of culture change.

Activity 10.2 Critical Thinking

Identify the quality standards that are relevant to your area of practice and how the KPIs they generate might align with the principles of culture change for people with dementia:

Principles of a culture change approach	Quality indicators that could be aligned	Examples of the quality indicator being achieved
Involvement of the person receiving care in directing the care they wish to receive		
Personalising the environment for the person with dementia. Ensuring there are artefacts that remind them of their past and their relationships		
Close relationships developed through informal and frequent interactions between staff, families and the person with dementia		
Staff empowerment – enabling staff to make the decisions to care flexibly and implement person-centred care		
Collaborative decision-making involving people with dementia, families and staff		
Systematic Quality Improvement		

Once we have decided on the KPIs that could be used to support the development of relationship-based approaches to care, we need next to consider a systematic way of implementing the change. In many studies, the use of iterative cycles such as the Plan–Do–Study–Act (PDSA) Cycle has been used to move through the change process

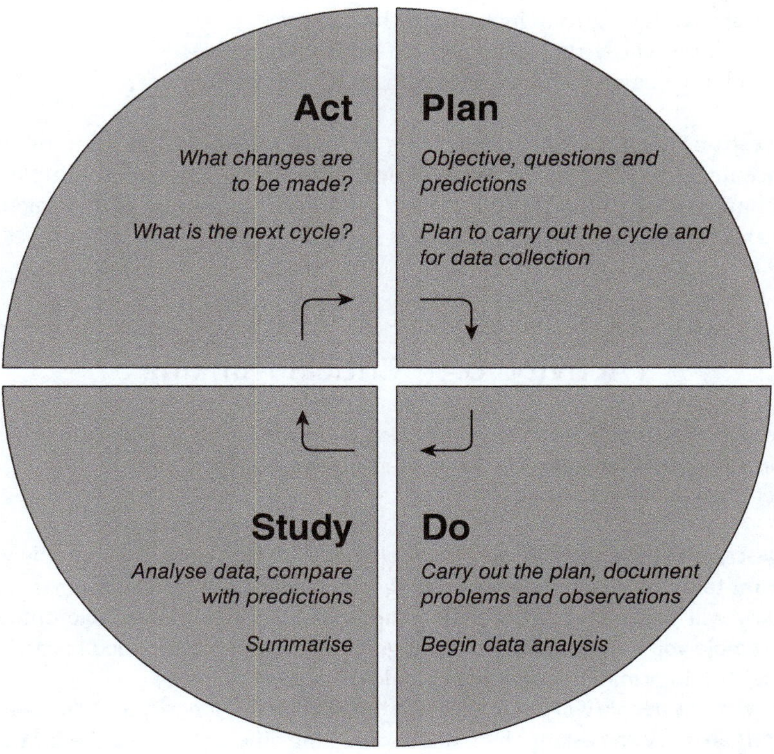

Figure 10.2 PDSA Cycle

(Figure 10.2). The PDSA is an action-oriented cycle that aims at testing out changes in the real world setting of practice on a small scale (Institute for Health Improvement, 2016) before implementing change more broadly. The PDSA Cycle is an effective way of learning if a new initiative may or may not work in a setting (Reed and Card, 2016). PDSA provides a simple structured approach to change and we will use this cycle to identify how we might embark on small-scale changes within the organisation in which we practise. The purpose of this will be to articulate the benefits of relationship-based approaches to care within the organisation. Such benefits have the potential to positively influence the experience of people with dementia, families and staff as well as the work environment through the teams and units providing care.

The PDSA Cycle may appear as a simple model but this does not necessarily mean it is easy to use (Reed and Card, 2016). Taylor et al. (2013) undertook a systematic review of PDSA projects and found that only two studies used the cycle effectively. However, PDSA is not intended to be used as a stand alone method since preparatory work is required to ensure the problem under review is framed and understood prior to embarking on the cycle (Reed and Card, 2016). To prepare for using the PDSA Cycle, the Institute for Health Improvement suggests three key questions be considered before embarking on change:

1. What are we trying to achieve with the change?
2. How will we know that change is an improvement?
3. What change can we make that will result in improvement?

These questions are a useful starting point to focus our minds on deciding what area of practice needs to be changed. We will now consider how we might implement one area of change in our practice to improve outcomes for people with dementia, their families and staff caring for them.

Activity 10.3 Critical Thinking

Using the activities completed so far in this book, choose one aspect of practice that you think would support the implementation of person-centred care (Figure 2.3).

Answer the following questions:

- Describe the change you want to implement – be **Specific** – for example you might want to support staff in implementing important details in care routines.
- How will you assess whether this happens? Identify a **Measurable** outcome – for example you might identify that biographical details are included in care plans and that this information is shared in handovers between shifts.
- How many people will you implement this change for? Identify an **Achievable** target – staff are busy and asking them to do something different will require time to achieve this, or else they might not engage with the change.
- Who will you involve in this project? Remember to be **Realistic** in terms of staff involvement – you will need people from different teams and possibly the informal gatekeepers and leaders too.
- How long will this project need? There needs to be a set **Time** for staff to achieve it, or else the momentum could be lost. The time also needs to be sufficient to enable measurable outcomes to occur.

You have now successfully developed a SMART objective for your project that will enable you to move into the planning stage.

Relationship-based approaches to care do not always have outcomes that are easy to measure. Nonetheless, it is an essential requirement that we identify measurable outcomes if we are to make the case for improving practice for people with dementia. Using an example from Chapter 6, you may wish to make a change to the physical environment to improve wayfinding thus enabling the person with dementia to access the toilet independently, reducing the incidence of incontinence in your facility. To achieve this, you might start with an environmental audit developed by the University of Stirling (see end of chapter) that identifies key environmental cues that would be helpful for the person with dementia. Alternatively, another starting point may be to take photographs of the environment before and after the proposed change (Roberts et al., 2015). A further outcome might be measured through an audit of the episodes of incontinence of people with dementia before and after the change to see if there has been any improvement. Using a further example from Chapter 7, you might wish to improve staff management of BPSD. This intervention might favour a staff education programme and could be assessed by looking at the incidence of behaviours that staff find challenging before and after the education programme. You might choose to do an audit of care records to assess the incidence of situations that staff documented as challenging; or you may choose to use an assessment tool to assess the behaviours of the person with dementia before and after the educational programme.

We have discussed the contribution of all stakeholders to the relationship in dementia care and a vital area of change management would be to capture the cognitive diversity of everyone who is likely to be involved in such change. This should include people with dementia and their families as they are most likely to be affected by the change and may be able to offer a differing perspective to support the identification of a shared solution. Practice scenario 10.1 identifies a change management project in residential care illustrating how the change was managed at each level of the organisation.

Practice scenario 10.1

Implementation of the ABLE model in residential aged care (Roberts et al., 2015)

This project implemented a Montessori approach in dementia care that promoted activity as part of the routines within the residential environment. Change was effected at three levels of the organisation:

Macro – Support from Board level and CEO for implementation of the new model alongside an agreement for training and development of staff: two days of dementia care training and two days of Montessori activity training, attended by all staff working in the Memory Support Unit (MSU).

Meso – A new position was created – 'Cognitive Rehabilitation Therapist (CRT)' – to undertake the leisure and lifestyle role. A part-time Dementia Consultant, with expertise in applying Montessori principles to dementia care, was also employed.

Micro – Residents and family members were engaged in the creation of biographical stories that resulted in visual displays of meaningful and personal items and/or written records of their life. Clinical assessment of residents identified their capacity for independence and how they might contribute to the community of the home using their cognitive and physical capabilities.

(Continued)

(Continued)

The change process

A project manager was employed. The CRT was a Montessori 'champion' for MSU staff on a day-to-day basis, and also facilitated the transitioning of new residents and their families from pre-admission to admission. Consultation and communication occurred between staff, residents, residents' families, the Nurse Unit Manager (NUM), CRT, and the project manager. The NUM also worked closely with the two local GPs to review residents' medications.

Planning a change from the outset is vital if we are going to be able to identify and measure the outcomes effectively. Many PDSA Cycles suffer from not spending sufficient time in the Planning phase, which often results in a poor understanding of resource requirements, or planning data collection that does not answer the questions posed (Reed and Card, 2016). Prior to implementation of a change, the 'who, what, where, when, and how' of implementation needs to be clearly articulated if you are to achieve the overall goal of the project. Use Activity 10.4 to develop a plan for your projected change.

Activity 10.4 Planning

The first stage is to identify what needs to be done and who is responsible for each action. It is helpful to break down the change into separate steps. The following table ensures you are also involving key stakeholders to include cognitive diversity in coming up with solutions at each level of the organisation. This also means including contributions from people with dementia and families.

Level of organisation	What needs to be done?	Who needs to be involved?	Who do we consult?	Who is responsible for leading?
Board level – mission statement, policies and procedures				
Middle management – agreement to work differently – team level decisions				
Direct care involving all staff, people with dementia and families				

The implementation phase of the project or the 'doing' part of the PDSA Cycle also includes collecting data for the 'Study' phase. This may include both quantitative data alongside qualitative data to explain why something may or may not have worked. A number of tools have also been developed for person-centred care in residential and acute care to consider the needs of people with dementia and how an organisation contributes to person-centred care (see Table 10.1). Ensuring the experience of the person with dementia and their families is captured requires careful consideration. This might be achieved through observations such as Dementia Care Mapping (Brooker and Surr, 2006; Roberts et al., 2015) or PIECE-Dem (Brooker and Latham, 2015).

The implementation phase of the PDSA Cycle influences the quality and quantity of data collected with a poor implementation phase impacting negatively on the subsequent study phase (Reed and Card, 2016). The PDSA Cycle can be used with other approaches and Practice Development is a helpful approach to engage staff who may be part of the change process. Practice Development methodology includes a facilitator who is responsible for introducing evidence-based thinking in a way that staff are able to engage with (Ryecroft-Malone, 2004). Having a facilitator present enables staff to use the presented evidence to identify solutions to issues they may be experiencing in practice. Practice Development might form part of the implementation phase as you bring staff

Table 10.1 Examples of evidence-based tools for person-centred care

Title	Authors	Description
The Tool for Understanding Residents' Needs as Individual Persons (TURNIP) in residential aged care	Edvardsson et al. (2011)	'The 39 item TURNIP conceptualised person-centred care into five dimensions: (1) the care environment, (2) staff members' attitudes towards dementia, (3) staff members' knowledge about dementia, (4) the care organisation and (5) the content of care provided.' (p. 2890)
The Person-Centred Care of Older People with Cognitive Impairment in Acute Care Scale (POPAC)	Edvardsson et al. (2013)	This tool is based on the following areas of best practice: 'recognizing cognitive impairment, consulting specialist expertise, using evidence-based care protocols or guidelines, making environmental adjustments, providing social enrichments, prioritizing staff continuity and close interactions, avoiding restraints, and individualizing care … developed into 21 items relating to best practice and eight items relating to staff attitudes towards older people with cognitive impairments.' (pp. 80–81)
Person-Centred Care Assessment Tool (P-CAT)	Edvardsson et al. (2010)	Measures person-centred environment to assess how organisational factors support or obstruct person-centred care: Subscale One: extent of personalising care Subscale Two: amount of organisational support Subscale Three: degree of environmental accessibility Correlating the subscales, this tool analyses the relationship between organisational support, environmental accessibility and the extent to which care is personalised.

together to discuss how the implementation phase is going and any resulting challenges. Kim Bezzant (2008) in the UK undertook a Practice Development project to support older patients with delirium and dementia in hospital (Practice scenario 10.2).

Practice scenario 10.2

Managing change in an acute hospital

This project had three phases that mapped to each level of the organisation:

> **Macro:** The development of clinical policies and guidelines supporting the care of people with cognitive impairment that were displaying unusual behaviours. This included the development of a pathway for people with dementia.
>
> **Meso:** The up-skilling of clinical teams in the care of people who exhibit unusual behaviours, through workshops which examined values, beliefs and practice alongside the challenges in managing behaviours and available support for these as appropriate.
>
> **Micro:** Working with direct care staff through practice-based facilitation and Action Learning Sets.

Source: Bezzant (2008: 144).

Action Learning Sets are groups of staff members who come together to consider an issue and devise subsequent strategies for dealing with that issue. The use of Action Learning Sets is a strategy that complements the view of organisations as CAS by providing an opportunity for staff to consider solutions collectively thus promoting self-organisation as staff produce new and creative ways of working. Schein (2010) suggests that staff need to feel psychologically safe as change is being implemented with opportunities for learning anxiety to be managed. Staff assimilating new concepts represents an integral part of the change process, supporting the embedding of the new behaviours. Action Learning Sets enable staff to come together in a supportive environment to discuss the change and how to manage unintended or unanticipated consequences. Using the safe environment of Action Learning Sets may contribute to re-framing the experience of staff to recognise the positive nature of the change. Using these ideas, implement the change you have identified and record your experience in Activity 10.5.

Activity 10.5 Doing

Once you have planned a change, you need to implement and reflect on the process. The process is the way the outcome has been achieved and may provide vital clues in implementing the change on a larger scale. There may be unintended consequences, both positive and negative, that were not foreseen. Capturing the process of change will support future evaluation of the change alongside the measurable outcomes. This in turn, will support the Study phase of the cycle.

Level of organisation	What was done?	How long did it take?	What were some of the issues experienced?	What worked well? Include evidence to support this
Board level – mission statement, policies and procedures				
Middle management – agreement to work differently – team level decisions				
Direct care involving all staff, people with dementia and families				

The Study phase of the PDSA Cycle may be overlooked in the desire to move forward with the Action phase of the Cycle. Giving insufficient time to the Study phase may restrict the learning of what worked and why, which will subsequently impact on the success of the change in the longer term (Reed and Card, 2016). The Study phase is where data collected in the Implementation phase are analysed and learning from the project communicated. Use Activity 10.6 to analyse the data collected from the project.

Activity 10.6 Study

Level of organisation	What were the outcomes measured?	What were the results?	What did the results tell us about the change?	How did this influence the experience of people with dementia, families and staff?
Board level – mission statement, policies and procedures				

(Continued)

(Continued)

Level of organisation	What were the outcomes measured?	What were the results?	What did the results tell us about the change?	How did this influence the experience of people with dementia, families and staff?
Middle management – agreement to work differently – team level decisions				
Direct care involving all staff, people with dementia and families				

The final phase of the PDSA Cycle is the Act phase where in light of the Study phase, decisions are made that can follow a number of paths. Two obvious paths might be either to sustain, embed or roll out the intervention, or to end the project without further investment. One of the benefits of the PDSA Cycle is discovering that some projects might not be realistic to solve in this way and knowing this avoids further investment and wasted effort from continuing work on the wrong problem. Alternatively, the Act phase may suggest that this project is a change that can be fully implemented and sustained. A key component of the Act phase is to consider the results in light of the broader theory or literature in the field. Failure to do this may risk overlooking barriers that may have been uncovered in similar projects (Reed and Card, 2016). Move on to Activity 10.7 to review your position in order to take the next steps.

Activity 10.7 Act

Level of organisation	What do we need to do next to Act on these results?	How could we improve in the next cycles?	What changes need to be made to the initial plan?	Who do we need to involve?
Board level – mission statement, policies and procedures				

Level of organisation	What do we need to do next to Act on these results?	How could we improve in the next cycles?	What changes need to be made to the initial plan?	Who do we need to involve?
Middle management – agreement to work differently – team level decisions				
Direct care involving all staff, people with dementia and families				

The 'Act' stage of the PDSA Cycle needs to consider how to embed the change if this is being done within one unit or how to move this change to other units.

If you feel you need to revisit this project, move back to the Planning phase and use the learning from this completed Cycle to move to another PDSA Cycle. Now that you have had experience of working through each aspect of this Cycle, you might consider other aspects of person-centred or relationship-centred care that you might implement using the same process.

Conclusion

Change management is often necessary within dementia care to ensure organisations are able to remain competitive, but considering relationships as a fundamental part of the organisational culture is helpful to promote relationship-based approaches to care. We have drawn on the leadership, culture and organisational change literature using the lens of Complex Adaptive Systems to examine a change management strategy to improve dementia care.

At the *macro* level of the organisation, language between policies, role descriptions/ person specifications needs to reflect person-centred and relationship-centred principles:

- Ensure the language of the vision and mission are replicated;
- Use person-centred language in defining the role and identifying the motivation of staff in taking on this role;
- Consider stakeholder feedback and include this in the role specifications to demonstrate inclusion of their perspectives;
- Look for the best evidence before making changes and involve managers in this process so they can see how the service philosophy is being shaped.

At the *meso* level of the organisation, relationship-oriented leadership and role modelling practices need to be implemented within and across teams:

- Promote cognitive diversity within teams;
- Enable frequent and informal interactions and so prompt problem solving and the development of shared understandings;
- Foster self-organisation as staff generate new patterns of working.

At the *micro* or direct care level, enable staff to engage and interact with people living with dementia, families and other staff:

- Actively encourage storytelling and capture this information in meaningful ways to support attention to significant details and engage the person with dementia in meaningful activity;
- Involve all stakeholders in decision-making, including people with dementia and their families to facilitate shared understandings;
- Anticipate how the environment may impact on the person with dementia and implement solutions to minimise adverse impacts.

Final reflections

Throughout this book, we have examined what is needed at each level of the organisation to facilitate relationship-based approaches to care. This final chapter has supported you in thinking about how you might assess the effectiveness of changes you may make and how such changes might influence each level of the organisation. The purpose of developing an organisational approach to dementia care is to improve the care and experience of the person with dementia, families and staff. We have explored a range of strategies that support staff in the implementation of relationship-based approaches along the continuum of care we discussed in Chapter 2 (Figure 2.5). Structured evaluation of new ways of working using QI methodology will demonstrate measurable outcomes and so ensure ongoing support for improving dementia care at each level of the organisation.

Further reading

Mind tools

A website with resources for the development of leadership and other skills for ongoing professional development. This is not specific to healthcare but draws on the wider management and leadership knowledge base. Available at: www.mindtools.com (accessed 27/01/17).

Institute for Health Improvement

This is a US-based organisation that provides tools and resources to support organisations worldwide in improving healthcare. Using the Science of Improvement it focuses on asking three specific questions and then using the PDSA Cycle to undertake experimental testing of innovation leading to rapid integration of successful projects. Available at: www.ihi.org/resources/Pages/HowtoImprove/default.aspx (accessed 27/01/17).

Examples of audit tools

The Dementia Services Centre, University of Stirling have developed a service that will audit your environment for accreditation. The audit tools are also available to purchase. Available at: http://dementia.stir.ac.uk/design/accreditation (accessed 27/01/17).

National Audit of Dementia, UK

The National Audit of Dementia is working with hospitals providing general acute inpatient services to measure criteria relating to care delivery, known to impact on people with dementia admitted to hospital. The first audit was completed in 2010, the second in 2012 with the third audit conducted 2016–2017. This website provides you with the background to the audit and reports from each round. The third round includes questionnaires to be handed to family caregivers and staff. Available at: www.rcpsych.ac.uk/workinpsychiatry/qualityimprovement/nationalclinicalaudits/dementia/nationalauditofdementia.aspx (accessed 27/01/17).

Round 3 Standards for the National Audit of Dementia as developed by the Royal College of Psychiatrists with input from the Royal College of Nursing (2015). Available at: www.rcpsych.ac.uk/pdf/CCQI%20NAD3%202015%20standards%20Aug%202015.pdf (accessed 27/01/17).

Conclusion: Making a difference

Relationships matter in dementia care and positive relationships with the person with dementia, their families and staff underpin every aspect of this care. Throughout this book we have examined the components of relationship-based approaches of care; we have discussed ways by which we could implement such practice across an organisation to improve the experience of the person with dementia, their families and supporters and staff who provide care. Dementia is affecting more people than ever before and as such all organisations now need to consider how to ensure positive outcomes for the person with dementia, their families and supporters as well as staff who provide care. Organisations are unable to provide effective dementia care unless the staff they employ are supported to work in a way that facilitates personal and responsive relationships. As dementia has been likened to a journey, this book has endeavoured to provide a 'road map' that provides organisations and the staff they support with tools by which to navigate this journey alongside the person with dementia and those who support them.

As with any journey, there is no single 'correct' way but rather a series of choices that reflect the needs and interests of those on that journey. We started with considering the myths associated with this journey. Interrogating such myths enables us to view the world from the perspective of the person with dementia; this is indeed the correct starting point for ensuring we implement person-centred and relationship-centred care. Myths beget stereotypes and stereotypes influence the decisions professionals make that enable or disable the person with dementia to realise their potential. We can choose to reframe such stereotypes through inclusive actions that value the stories shared by the person with dementia, their families and supporters. Reframing begins with understanding how the sharing of stories and anecdotes contributes to the building of relationships through which we develop strategies to improve care and support for people with dementia and those who support them. The underpinning respectful communication of relationship-based approaches to care ensures we value the person with dementia and the unique life experience they bring to their dementia journey. Respectful communication and valuing what is significant in the person with dementia's life lays an effective foundation for cultural responsiveness in relationship-based approaches to care.

Relationship-based approaches summarise a continuum of care that focuses on the value of relationships between the person with dementia, those who support them and staff (Figure C.1). Recognising that staff adopt different practices depending on the constraints at the time enables us to adopt a more flexible position between individualised, person-centred and relationship-centred care as

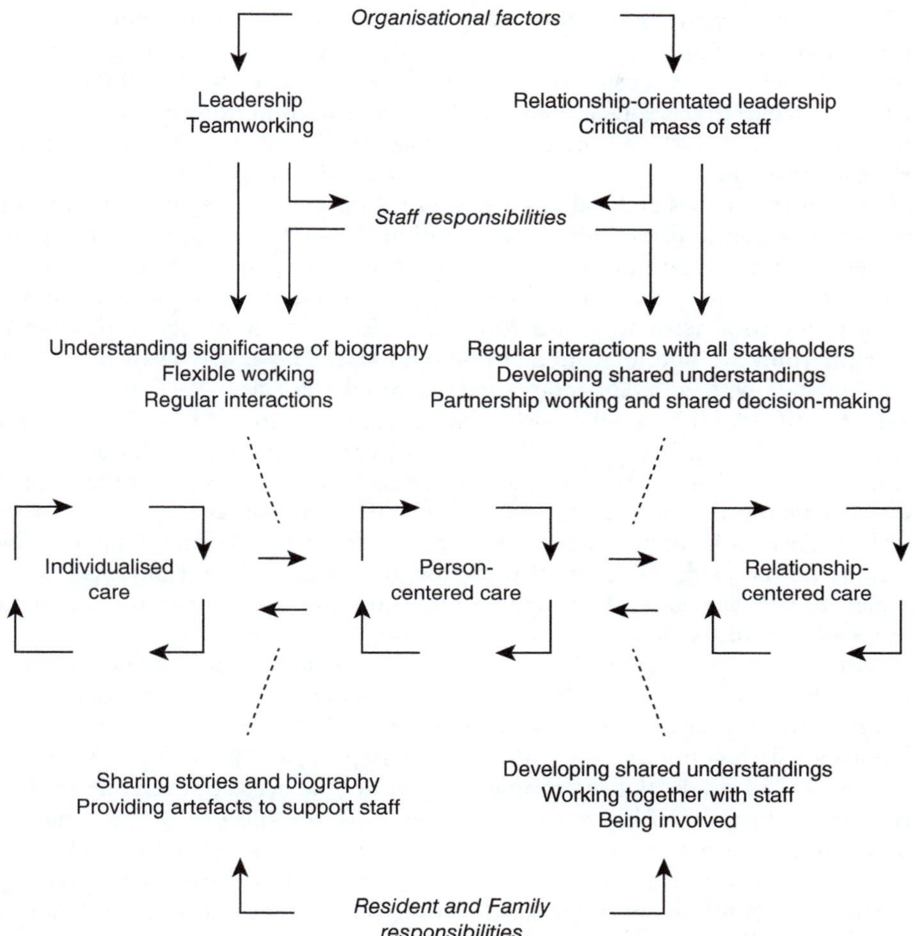

Figure C.1

circumstances evolve. This means that when there are situations where person-centred care may not be possible, then individualised care becomes the acceptable default position, rather than a focus on the task. The idea of a continuum reflects that people can also move from individualised to person-centred and on to relationship-centred care. To facilitate movement implies flexibility and each level of the organisation needs to be supportive of this flexibility if relationship-based approaches to care are to be effectively implemented in practice.

Relationship-based approaches to care begin with understanding how life experience and relationship to community shapes the person. Individualised care provides a starting point by asking about the life experience of a person and the choices they wish to have in their day-to-day life. The key distinction in moving to person-centred care is finding out 'why' this experience is significant to this person and how this experience actively shapes the decisions this person is now making.

The value of biography shared through stories and anecdotes is recognised and this information is then used to shape the care for the person with dementia. Leadership by example, where care is role modelled across the team, is a key factor in supporting staff in moving to person-centred care. Communication through frequent and informal interactions where stories and anecdotes are shared provides the opportunity for personalised and responsive actions. Involving all stakeholders, i.e. the person with dementia, families and staff, in decisions promotes diversity of perspective thus developing shared understandings. Recognition of the contributions of the person with dementia and their family are pivotal in staff moving along the continuum.

In returning to the metaphor of this book as a 'road map', there being many ways in journeying to a destination, for some of us it is not about the destination but rather the route we take that needs to be the focus. This is a relevant focus when involving staff with different motivations in providing care. Developing a critical mass of staff adopting a relationship-based approach to care is vital to ensure consistency of care across teams. Working with the staff's mental models of care through facilitated workshops is one route that this journey might take. Equally, there may be more structured approaches to staff education and training that may be taken. This book has provided a number of evidence-based examples upon which decisions can be made. When staff recognise and value the contributions made by the person with dementia, their families and supporters, this forms the foundation upon which shared understandings may develop.

Relationship-centred care (RCC) provides the vehicle through which we value these multiple perspectives, develop shared understandings and subsequently consider how to meet everyone's needs within the relationship. RCC focuses on the relationship with community and this book has provided examples of where this might be used in residential environments to ensure the needs of everyone are being met. There is further work needed to consider RCC in respect to cultures that have a more collective focus and how RCC might be implemented for people with dementia who continue to reside within their communities. Partnership working is central to the implementation of RCC as everyone's needs within the relationship are recognised. Working in partnership is the first step in ensuring there is a diversity of perspectives contributing to shared decision-making.

The destination and even the journey towards the implementation of relationship-based approaches to dementia care will be influenced by the organisation. Within each level of the organisation, we have examined the mechanisms that can be used to positively influence this journey. The value of informal interactions that promote cognitive diversity in decision-making cannot be underestimated in delivering relationship-based approaches to care. Frequent interactions that encourage problem solving, followed by a flexible response as staff then self-organise to implement the solution, promote new behaviours and provide staff with the flexibility to meet the needs of everyone within the relationship. Relationship-oriented leadership in this context is paramount where individuals who can be flexible in their style of leadership to meet changing needs with changing leadership styles are needed. Quality Improvement (QI) methodology facilitates a structured approach when we implement change and enables us to identify appropriate outcomes on which to build sustainability. QI needs to be an integral part of our journey but as with the rest of the road map, there is no one way of using this. QI can support us in evaluating how we have journeyed and whether we have reached our first destination. It can also provide support for other parts of the organisation in how they may choose to journey towards providing relationship-based approaches to dementia care. Our role within QI is to consider how we might operate as both a leader and a manager and to realise improved outcomes in the care of those with dementia and their families.

This leaves us with the question: who will take the first step in promoting improved care for the person with dementia and those who support them? The first step requires leadership in communicating the vision; the second step is management leading towards sustainable change; and the third step calls for motivation to make a difference. I hope this person will be you and that this book provides you with the support to make a difference to the lives of people with dementia, their families and supporters within the organisation in which you practise.

References

Aalten, P., de Vugt, M.E., Lousberg, R., et al. (2003) Behavioral problems in dementia: a factor analysis of the neuropsychiatric inventory. *Dementia and Geriatric Cognitive Disorders*, 15: 99–105.

Aalten, P., de Vugt, M., Jaspers, N., Jolles, J. and Verhey, F. (2005a) The course of neuropsychiatric symptoms in dementia. Part I: findings from the two-year longitudinal Maasbed study. *International Journal of Geriatric Psychiatry*, 20: 523–530.

Aalten, P., de Vugt, M., Jaspers, N., Jolles, J. and Verhey, F. (2005b) The course of neuropsychiatric symptoms in dementia. Part II: relationships among behavioural sub-syndromes and the influence of clinical variables. *International Journal of Geriatric Psychiatry*, 20: 531–536.

Albert, M.S., DeKosky, S.T., Dickson, D., et al. (2011) The diagnosis of mild cognitive impairment due to Alzheimer's disease: recommendations from the National Institute on Aging and Alzheimer's Association workgroup. *Alzheimer's Dementia*, 7(3): 270–279.

Alexander, G., Rantz, M.J., Skubic, M., Koopman, R., Phillips, L., Guevara, R. and Miller, S. (2011) Evolution of an early illness warning system to monitor frail elders in independent living. *Journal of Healthcare Engineering*, 2: 259–286.

Algase, D.L., Beck, C., Kolanowski, A., et al. (1966) Need-driven dementia compromised behavior: an alternative view of disruptive behavior. *American Journal of Alzheimer's Disease*, 11: 10–19.

Allen, J., Oyebode, J. and Allen, J. (2009) Having a father with young onset dementia. The impact on well-being of young people. *Dementia*, 8(4): 455–480.

Alzheimer's Australia (2015) *About Dementia,* Fact sheet: Available at: https://fightdementia.org.au/national/about-dementia/types-of-dementia (accessed 09/01/16).

Alzheimer's Disease International and World Health Organization (2012) *Dementia: A Public Health Priority*. Geneva, Switzerland: World Health Organization. Available at: www.who.int/mental_health/publications/dementia_report_2012/en/ (accessed 10/01/16).

Alzheimer's Society (2013) *End of Life Care*, Fact sheet 531LP. Available at: www.alzheimers.org.uk/site/scripts/documents_info.php?documentID=2709 (accessed 22/08/16).

Alzheimer's Society (2014) *Dementia UK*, second edition. Available at: www.youngdementiauk.org/sites/default/files/Dementia_UK_Second_edition_-_Overview.pdf (accessed 22/08/16).

Alzheimer's Society (2015) *What is Mild Cognitive Impairment?* Fact sheet. Available at: www.alzheimers.org.uk/site/scripts/documents_info.php?documentID=120 (accessed 08/01/16).

Anderson, R.A. and McDaniel, Jr., R.R. (1998) Intensity of registered nurse participation in nursing home decision making. *Gerontologist*, 38(1): 90–100.

Anderson, R.A., Issel, L.M. and McDaniel, Jr., R.R. (2003) Nursing homes as complex adaptive systems: relationship between management practice and resident outcomes. *Nursing Research*, 52(1): 12–21.

Anderson, R.A., Ammarell, N., et al. (2005a) Quality improvement in long-term care: the power of relationships for high-quality long-term care. *Journal of Nursing Care Quality*, 20(2): 103–106.

Anderson, R.A., Ammarell, N., et al (2005b) Nursing assistant mental models, sense making, care actions, and consequences for nursing home residents. *Qualitative Health Research*, 15(8): 1006–1021.

Anderson, R.A., Plowman, D., Corazzini, K., Hsieh, P.-C., Su, H.-F., Landerman, L.R. and McDaniel, R.R. (2013) Participation in decision making as a property of complex adaptive systems: developing and testing a measure. *Nursing Research and Practice*, 1–16.

Association for Dementia Studies (2010) 'It's what you do and the way that you do it'. A report on Howbury Lodge Day Centre. Friends of the Elderly, Malvern Worcesrshire. Available at: www.worcester.ac.uk/documents/Howbury_Evaluation_Report.pdf (accessed 21/01/16).

Aud, M.A. (2004) Dangerous wandering: elopements of older adults with dementia from long-term care facilities. *American Journal of Alzheimers Disease and Other Dementias*, 19(6): 361–368.

Australian Institute of Health and Welfare (2012) *Dementia in Australia*. Available at: www.aihw.gov.au/WorkArea/DownloadAsset.aspx?id=10737422943 (accessed 10/01/16).

Baker, C.J. (2009) Introducing PEARL: rewarding good practice in dementia care. *Journal of Dementia Care*, 17(4): 31–34.

Baker, C.J. (2015) The PEARL programme: caring for adults living with dementia. *Nursing Standard*, 30(5): 46–51.

Bakker, C., e Vugt, M., an Vliet, D., Verhey, F., Pijnenburg, Y., Vernooij-Dassen, M. and Koopmans, R. (2013) The use of formal and informal care in early onset dementia: results from the NeedYD Study. *The American Journal of Geriatric Psychiatry*, 21(1): 37–45.

Banaszak-Holl, J., Castle, N.G., Lin, M. and Spreitzer, G. (2013) An assessment of cultural values and resident-centred culture change in US nursing facilities. *Health Care Management Review*, 38(4): 295–305.

Bangar, S., Mountain, G. and Cudd, P. (2015) Assistive Technology: creating and engaging collaborative communities. *Studies in Health Technology and Informatics*, 217: 730–735.

Barnes, D. and Yaffe, K. (2011) The projected impact of risk factor reduction on Alzheimer's Disease prevalence. *Lancet, Neurology*, 10(9): 819–828.

Barrett, C., Whyte, C., Leonard, W. and Comfort, J. (2014) No need to straighten up: discrimination, depression and anxiety in older lesbian, gay, bisexual, transgender and intersex Australians. Australian Research Centre in Sex, Health and Society. Melbourne: La Trobe University. Available at: www.beyondblue.org.au/docs/default-source/research-project-files/bw0263-no-need-to-straighten-up---full-report---pdf.pdf?sfvrsn=2 (accessed 14/09/16).

Barrett, C., Crameri, P., Lambourne, S. and Latham, J.R. (2015) 'We are still gay…': the needs of LGBT Australians with dementia. *Australasian Journal of Dementia Care*. Available at: http://journalofdementiacare.com/we-are-still-gay-the-needs-of-lgbt-australians-with-dementia/ (accessed 1/11/16).

Basu, R., Hochhalter, A. and Stevens, A. (2015) The impact of the REACH II intervention on caregivers' perceived health. *Journal of Applied Gerontology*, 34(5): 590–608.

Bauer, M. (2006) Collaboration and control: nurses' constructions of the role of family in nursing home care. *Journal of Advanced Nursing*, 54(1): 45–52.

Bauer, M., Fetherstonhaugh, D., Nay, R., Tarzia, L. Nay, R., Wellman, D. and Beattie, E. (2013a) 'I always look under the bed for a man'. Needs and barriers to the expression of sexuality in residential aged care: the views of residents with and without dementia. *Psychology & Sexuality*, 4(3): 296–309.

Bauer, M., Fetherstonhaugh, D., Nay, R., Tarzia, L. and Beattie, E. (2013b) Sexuality Assessment Tool (SexAT) for residential aged care facilities. Available at: www.agedcare.

org.au/publications/agendas-docs-images/sexuality-assessment-tool-sexat-for-residential-aged-care-facilities (accessed 30/09/16).

Bauer, M., Fetherstonhaugh, D., Nay, R., Tarzia, L. and Beattie, E. (2014a) Supporting residents' expression of sexuality: the initial construction of a sexuality assessment tool for residential aged care facilities. *BMC Geriatrics*, 14: 82.

Bauer, M., Fetherstonhaugh, D., Nay, R., Tarzia, L., Nay, R., Wellman, D. and Beattie, E. (2014b) 'We need to know what's going on': views of family members toward the sexual expression of people with dementia in residential aged care. *Dementia*, 13(5): 571–585.

Bell, G. (2014) *Changing Care Culture: Exploring the Relationship between Employee Beliefs, Affective Commitment and Job Satisfaction Following a Change from Traditional to Person-Centred Care in Two Irish Nursing Homes*. National College of Ireland.

Belle, S.H., Burgio, L., Burns, R., Coon, D., Czaja, S.J., Gallagher-Thompson, D. and Zhang, S. (2006) Enhancing the quality of life of dementia caregivers from different ethnic or racial groups: a randomized, controlled trial. *Annals of Internal Medicine*, 145: 727–738.

Bellot, J.L. (2007) A descriptive study of nursing home organizational culture, work environment and culture change from the perspectives of licensed nurses. PhD thesis, University of Pennsylvania.

Bemelmans, R., Gelderblom, G.J., Jonker, P. and de Witte, L. (2012) Socially assistive robots in elderly care: a systematic review into effects and effectiveness. *Journal of the American Medical Directors Association*, 13: 114–120.

Ben-Tovim, D., Bassham, J., Bennett, D., Dougherty, M., Martin, M., O'Neill, S., Sincock, J. and Szwarcbord, M. (2008) Redesigning care at the Flinders Medical Centre: clinical process redesign using 'lean thinking'. *Medical Journal Australia*, 188(6): S27–S31.

Bezzant, K. (2008) Practice development: providing benefits for both managers and older patients with delirium and dementia. *Journal of Nursing Management*, 16: 141–146.

Bharucha, A., Anand,V., Forlizzi, J. et al. (2009) Intelligent assistive technology applications to dementia care: current capabilities, limitations, and future challenges. *American Journal Geriatiric Psychiatry*, 17(2): 88–104.

Biundo, S., Höller, D., Schattenberg, B. and Bercher, P. (2016) Companion-technology: an overview. *Künstliche Intelligenz*, 30: 11–20.

Boal, K. and Schultz, P. (2007) Storytelling, time, and evolution: the role of strategic leadership in complex adaptive systems. *The Leadership Quarterly*, 18: 411–428.

Borbasi, S., Jones, J., Lockwood, C. and Emden, C. (2006) Health professionals' perspectives of providing care to people with dementia in the acute setting: toward better practice. *Geriatric Nursing*, 27(5): 300–308.

Brady Germain, P. and Cummings, G. (2010) The influence of nursing leadership on nurse performance: a systematic literature review. *Journal of Nursing Management*, 18: 425–439.

Bramble, M., Moyle, W. and Shum, D. (2011) A quasi-experimental design trial exploring the effect of a partnership intervention on family and staff well-being in long-term dementia care. *Aging & Mental Health*, 15(8): 995–1007.

British Standard Institution (BSI) (2010) PAS 800 Use of Dementia Care Mapping for improved person-centred care in a care provider organisation. Available at: http://shop.bsigroup.com/en/ProductDetail/?pid=000000000030186216 (accessed 21/01/16).

Brodaty, H. and Arasaratnam, C. (2012) Meta-analysis of nonpharmacological interventions for neuropsychiatric symptoms of dementia. *American Journal of Psychiatry*, 169: 946–953.

Brodaty, H. and Donkin, M. (2009) Family caregivers of people with dementia. *Dialogues of Clinical Neuroscience*, 11: 217–228.

Brooker, D. (2004) What is Person-Centred Care for people with dementia? *Reviews in Clinical Gerontology*, 13: 215–222.

Brooker, D. and Latham, I. (2015) *Person-Centred Dementia Care: Making Services Better with the VIPS Framework* (second edition). London: Jessica Kingsley Publishers.

Brooker, D. and Surr, C. (2006) Dementia Care Mapping (DCM): initial validation of DCM 8 in UK field trials. *International Journal of Geriatric Psychiatry*, 21(11): 1018–1025.

Brooker, D. and Woolley, R. (2007) Enriching opportunities for people living with dementia: the development of a blueprint for a sustainable activity-based model of care. *Aging and Mental Health*, 11(4): 371–383.

Brooker, D., Woolley, R. and Lee, D. (2007) Enriching opportunities for people living with dementia in nursing homes: an evaluation of a multi-level activity-based model of care. *Aging and Mental Health*, 11(4): 361–370.

Brooker, D., La Fontaine, J., Evans, S., Bray, J. and Saad, K. (2014) Public health guidance to facilitate timely diagnosis of dementia: ALzheimer's COoperative Valuation in Europe (ALCOVE) recommendations. *International Journal of Geriatric Psychiatry*, 29: 682–693.

Brown, J., Davies, S. and Nolan, M. (2001) Who's the expert? Redefining lay and professional relationships. In M. Nolan, S. Davies and G. Grant (eds), *Working with Older People and their Families*. Buckingham: Open University Press. pp.19–32.

Brown Wilson, C. (2007) Exploring relationships in care homes. Unpublished thesis, University of Sheffield.

Brown Wilson, C. (2009) Developing community in care homes through a relationship-centred approach. *Health and Social Care in the Community*, 17(2): 177–186.

Brown Wilson, C. (2012) *Caring for Older People: A Shared Approach*. London: Sage.

Brown Wilson, C. and Davies, S. (2009) Using relationships in care homes to develop relationship centred care: the contribution of staff. *Journal of Clinical Nursing*, 18: 1746–1755.

Brown Wilson, C., Davies, S. and Nolan, M.R. (2009) Developing relationships in care homes: the contribution of staff, residents and families. *Ageing and Society*, 29(7): 1041–1063.

Brown Wilson, C., Swarbrick, C., Pilling, M. and Keady, J. (2013) The senses in practice: enhancing the quality of care for residents with dementia in care homes. *Journal of Advanced Nursing*, 69(1): 70–77.

Bruen, W. and Howe, A. (2009) Respite care for people living with dementia. 'It's more than just a short break'. Alzheimer's Australia. Available at: www.fightdementia.org.au/files/20090500_Nat_NP_17RespCarePplLivDem.pdf (accessed 21/06/16).

Bryden, C. (2002) A person-centred approach to counselling, psychotherapy and rehabilitation of people diagnosed with dementia in the early stages. *Dementia*, 1(2): 141–156.

Bryden, C. (2015) *Before I Forget: How I Survived Being Diagnosed with Younger-Onset Dementia at 46*. Australia: Penguin.

Bunn, F., Goodman, C., Pinkney, E. and. Drennan, V. (2016) Specialist nursing and community support for the carers of people with dementia living at home: an evidence synthesis. *Health and Social Care in the Community*, 24(1): 48–67.

Burgio, L.D., Collins, I.B., Schmid, B., Wharton, T., McCallum, D. and Decoster, J. (2009) Translating the REACH caregiver intervention for use by area agency on aging personnel: the REACH OUT program. *Gerontologist*, 49(1): 103–16.

Burns, K., Jayasinha, R., Tsang, R. and Brodaty, H. (2012) *Behaviour Management – A Guide to Good Practice*. Dementia Collaborative Research Centre. NSW. Available at: http://dbmas.org.au/uploads/resources/DBMAS_Guide_21_05_12.for_USB_pdf.pdf (accessed 05/08/16).

Carbonneau, H., Caron, C. and Desrosiers, J. (2010) Development of a conceptual framework of positive aspects of caregiving in dementia. *Dementia*, 9(3): 327–353.

The Carer Recognition Act, 2010. Available at: www.gov.uk/government/uploads/system/uploads/attachment_data/file/268684/Factsheet_8_update__tweak_.pdf (accessed 09/09/16).

Carteret, M. (2010) *Dimensions of Culture: Culturally Responsive Care*. Available at: www.dimensionsofculture.com/2010/10/576/ (accessed 14/09/16).

Cavallo, F., Aquilano, M. and Arvati, M. (2015) An ambient assisted living approach in designing domiciliary services combined with innovative technologies for patients with Alzheimer's Disease: a case study. *American Journal of Alzheimer's Disease & Other Dementias*, 30(1): 69–77.

Cerejeira, J., Lagarto, L. and Mukaetova-Ladinska, E. (2012) Behavioral and psychological symptoms of dementia. *Frontiers in Neurology*, 3(73): 1–21.

Chaffee, M. and McNeill, M. (2007) A model of nursing as a complex adaptive system. *Nurings Outlook*, 55(5): 232–241.

Chalfont, G.E. (2006) Connection to nature at the building edge: towards a therapeutic architecture for dementia care environments. PhD thesis. Available at: www.chalfontdesign.com/media/CHALFONT%20PhD%20May%202006.pdf (accessed 1/11/16).

Chater, K. and Hughes, N. (2012) Strategies to deliver dementia training and education in the acute hospital setting. *Journal of Research in Nursing*, 18(6): 578–593.

Chen, D., Ashok, J., Bharucha, M.D. and Wactlar, H.D. (2007) *Intelligent Video Monitoring to Improve Safety of Older Persons*. 29th Annual International Conference of the IEEE Engineering in Medicine and Biology Series, 22–26 Aug.

Chenoweth, L., King, M.T., Jeon, Y.H., Brodaty, H., Stein-Parbury, J., Norman, R., Has, M. and Luscombe, G. (2009) Caring for Aged Dementia Care Resident Study (CADRES) of person-centred care, dementia-care mapping, and usual care in dementia: a cluster-randomised trial. *Lancet Neurology*, 8: 317–325.

Chenoweth, L., Forbes, I., Fleming, R., King, M., Stein-Parbury, J., Luscombe, G., Kenny, P., Jeon, Y.-H., Haas, M. and Brodaty, H. (2014) PerCEN: a cluster randomized controlled trial of person-centred residential care and environment for people with dementia. *International Psychogeriatrics*, 26(7): 1147–1160.

Cheung, K., Lau, B., Wong, P., Leung, A., Lou, V., Chan, G. and Schulz, R. (2015) Multicomponent intervention on enhancing dementia caregiver well-being and reducing behavioral problems among Hong Kong Chinese: a translational study based on REACH II. *International Journal of Geriatric Psychiatry*, 30: 460–469.

Cilliers, P. (1998) *Complexity and Post Modernism: Understanding Complex Systems*. London: Routledge.

Clemerson, G., Walsh, S. and Isaac, C. (2014) Towards living well with young onset dementia: an exploration of coping from the perspective of those diagnosed. *Dementia*, 13(4): 451–466.

Clissett, P., Porock, D., Harwood, R.H. and Gladman, J.R.F. (2013a) The responses of healthcare professionals to the admission of people with cognitive impairment to acute hospital settings: an observational and interview study. *Journal of Clinical Nursing*, 23: 1820–1829.

Clissett, P., Porock, D., Harwood, R.H. and Gladman, J.R.F. (2013b) The challenges of achieving person-centred care in acute hospitals: a qualitative study of people with dementia and their families. *International Journal of Nursing Studies*, 50: 1495–1503.

Colon-Emeric, C., Lekan-Rutledge, D., Utley-Smith, Q., Ammarell, N., Bailey, D., Piven, M., Corazzini, K. and Anderson, R.A (2006) Connection, regulation, and care. *Health Care Management Review,* 31(4): 337–346.

Connor, M. and Pakora, J. (2007) *Coaching and Mentoring at Work: Developing Effective Practice*. Berkshire: Open University Press.

Cooke, M., Moyle, W., Venturato, L., Walters, C. and Kinnane, J. (2014) Evaluation of an education intervention to implement a capability model of dementia care. *Dementia*, 13(5): 613–625.

Davies, S. (2003) Creating community: the basis for caring partnerships in nursing homes. In M.R. Nolan, U. Lundh, G. Grant and J. Keady (eds), *Partnerships in Family Care*. Maidenhead: Open University Press.

Davies, S. and Nolan, M.R. (2004) 'Making the move': relatives' experiences of the transition to a care home. *Health and Social Care in the Community,* 12(6): 517–526.

Davis, S., Byers, S., Nay, R. and Koch, S. (2009) Guiding design of dementia friendly environments in residential care settings. *Dementia*, 8: 185.

Department of Health (2009) *Living Well with Dementia*. Available at: www.gov.uk/government/publications/living-well-with-dementia-a-national-dementia-strategy (accessed 10/01/16).

Department of Health (2011) *Whole System Demonstrator Programme*. Available at : www.gov.uk/government/uploads/system/uploads/attachment_data/file/215264/dh_131689.pdf (accessed 10/09/16).

Department of Health (2013) The Care Act, 2014. Available at: www.carersact.org.au/Assets/Files/fed_national-carers-strategy_2011.pdf (accessed 09/09/16).

Dewing, J. (2004) Concerns relating to the application of frameworks to promote person-centredness in nursing older people. *International Journal of Older People Nursing*, 13(3a): 39–44.

Dewing, J. and Dijk, S. (2016) What is the current state of care for older people with dementia in general hospitals? A literature review. *Dementia*, 15(1): 106–124.

Doll, G.M.A. (2003) An exploratory study of the process of culture change in three Kansas nursing homes. PhD thesis. Kansas State University.

Dooley, K. (1997) A Complex Adaptive Systems model of organization change. *Nonlinear Dynamics, Psychology, and Life Sciences*, 1(1): 69–97.

Downs, M. and Bowers, B. (2014) *Excellence in Dementia Care* (second edition). Milton Keynes: Open University Press.

Drentea, P., Clay, O., Roth, D. and Mittelman, M. (2006) Predictors of improvement in social support: five-year effects of a structured intervention for caregivers of spouses with Alzheimer's disease. *Social Science & Medicine*, 63: 957–967.

Edvardsson, D. and Nay, R. (2009) Acute care and older people: challenges and ways forward. *Australian Journal of Advanced Nursing*, 27(2): 63–69.

Edvardsson, D., Fetherstonhaugh, D. and Nay, R. (2010) Promoting a continuation of self and normality: person-centred care as described by people with dementia, their family members and aged care staff. *Journal of Clinical Nursing*, 19: 2611–2618.

Edvardsson, D., Fetherstonhaugh, D. and Nay, R. (2011) The Tool for Understanding Residents' Needs as Individual Persons (TURNIP): construction and initial testing. *Journal of Clinical Nursing*, 20: 2890–2896.

Edvardsson, D., Nilsson, A., Fetherstonhaugh, D., Nay, R. and Crowe S. (2013) The person-centred care of older people with cognitive impairment in acute care scale (POPAC). *Journal of Nursing Management*, 21: 79–86.

Engstrom, M., Lindqvist, R., Ljunngren, B. and Carlsson, M. (2009) Staff members' perceptions of an ICT support package in dementia care during the process of implementation. *Journal of Nursing Management*, 17: 781–789.

Evans, N., Carey-Smith, B. and Orpwood, R. (2011) Using smart technology in an enabling way: a review of using technology to support daily life for a tenant with moderate dementia. *British Journal of Occupational Therapy*, 74(5): 249–253.

Exley, C., Bamford, C., Hughes, J. and Robinson, L. (2009) Advance care planning: an opportunity for person-centred care for people living with dementia. *Dementia*, 8(3): 419–424.

Fleming, R., Goodenough, B., Low, L.-F., Chenoweth, L. and Brodaty, H. (2016) The relationship between the quality of the built environment and the quality of life of people with dementia in residential care. *Dementia*, 15(4): 663–680.

Frank, L., Lloyd, A., Flynn, J.A., Kleinman, L., Matza, L.S., Margolis, M.K., et al. (2006) Impact of cognitive impairment on mild dementia patients and mild cognitive impairment patients and their informants. *International Psychogeriatrics*, 18: 151–162.

Fujinami, T., Miura, M., Takatsuka, R. and Sugihara, T. (2011) A study of long term tendencies in residents' activities of daily living at a group home for people with dementia using RFID slippers. *Proceedings of the 9th International Conference on Smart Homes and Health Telematics*, ICOST.

Galambos, C., Skubic, M., Wang, S. and Rantz, M. (2013) Management of dementia and depression utilizing in-home passive sensor data. *Gerontechnology: International Journal on the Fundamental Aspects of Technology to Serve the Ageing Society*, 11: 457–468.

Garand, L., Lingler, J., O'Connor, K. and Dew, A. (2009) Diagnostic labels, stigma, and participation in research related to dementia and mild cognitive impairment. *Research in Gerontological Nursing*, 2(2): 112–121.

Gaugler, J.G., Roth, D.L., Haley, W.E. and Mittelman, M.S. (2008) Can counseling and support reduce burden and depressive symptoms in caregivers of people with Alzheimer's disease during the transition to institutionalization? Results from the New York University caregiver intervention study. *Journal of the American Geriatrics Society*, 56: 421–428.

Gerdner, L.A., Buckwalter, K.C. and Reed, D. (2002) Impact of a psychoeducational intervention on caregiver response to behavioral problems. *Nursing Research*, 51: 363–374.

Gilliard, J. and Marshall, M. (eds) (2012) *Transforming the Quality of Life for People with Dementia through Contact with the Natural World*. London: Jessica Kingsley.

Gladman, J., Porock, D., Griffiths, A., Clissett, P., Harwood, R., Knight, A., Jurgens, F., Jones, R., Schneider, J. and Kearney, F. (2012) *Care of Older People with Cognitive Impairment in General Hospitals*. Available at: www.netscc.ac.uk/hsdr/files/project/SDO_FR_08-1809-227_V01.pdf (accessed 20/07/16).

Godwin, B. (2012) The ethical evaluation of assistive technology for practitioners: a checklist arising from a participatory study with people with dementia, family and professionals. *Journal of Assistive Technologies*, 6(2): 123–135.

Goffman, E. (1963) *Stigma: Notes on the Management of Spoiled Identity*. Englewood Cliffs, NJ: Prentice Hall.

Goleman, D. (2000) Leadership that gets results. *Harvard Business Review*. March–April: 79–90.

Graham, N., Lindesay, J., Katona, C., Bertolote, J.M., Camus, V., Copeland, J.R., et al. (2003) Reducing stigma and discrimination against older people with mental disorders: a technical consensus statement. *International Journal of Geriatric Psychiatry*, 18: 670–678.

Greiner, C., Makimoto, K., Suzuki, M., Yamakawa, M. and Ashida, N. (2007) Feasibility study of the integrated circuit tag monitoring system for dementia residents in Japan. *American Journal of Alzheimer's Disease and Other Dementias*, 22: 129–136.

Griffin, J., Meis, L., Greer, N., MacDonald, R., Jensen, A., Rutks, I., Carlyle, M. and Wilt, T. (2015) Effectiveness of caregiver interventions on patient outcomes in adults with dementia or Alzheimer's Disease: a systematic review. *Gerontology & Geriatric Medicine*, 1– 17.

Grünerbl, A., Bahle, G., Lukowicz, P. and Hanser, F. (2011) Using indoor location to assess the state of dementia patients: results and experience report from a long term, real world study. Seventh International Conference on Intelligent Environments. IEEE, 32–39.

Haley, W.E., Bergman, E.J., Roth, D.L., McVie, T., Gaugler, J.E. and Mittelman, M.S. (2008) Long-term effects of bereavement and caregiver intervention on dementia care. *The Gerontologist*, 48: 732–740.

Han, J.W., Kim, T.H., Lee, S.B., et al. (2012) Predictive validity and diagnostic stability of mild cognitive impairment subtypes. *Alzheimer's Dementia*, 8(6): 553–559.

Hanser, F., Grünerbl, A., Rodegast, C. and Lukowicz, P. (2008) Design and real life deployment of a pervasive monitoring system for dementia patients. In: Proceedings of the 2nd International Conference on Pervasive Computing Technologies for Healthcare.

Heinrich, S., Berwig, M., Simon, S., Jänichen, J., Hallensleben, N., Nickel, W., Hinz, A., Brähler, E. and Gertz, H. (2014) German adaptation of the Resources for Enhancing Alzheimer's Caregiver Health II: study protocol of a single-centred, randomized controlled trial. *BMC Geriatrics*, 14: 21.

Hersey, P., Blanchard, K. and Johnson, D. (2001) *Management of Organisational Behaviour: Leading Human Resources*. New Jersey: Prentice Hall, Inc.

Hertzberg, A., Ekman, S.L. and Axelsson, K. (2003) 'Relatives are a resource, but…': Registered nurses' views and experiences of relatives of residents in nursing homes. *Journal of Clinical Nursing*, 12(3): 431– 441.

Hirschman, K.B., Joyce, C.M., James, B.D., Xie, S.X. and Karlawish, J.H. (2005) Do Alzheimer's disease patients want to participate in a treatment decision, and would their carers let them? *The Gerontologist*, 45(3): 381–388.

Holmes, D., Teresi, J.A., Ramirez, M., Ellis, J., Eimicke, J., Jian, K., et al. (2007) An evaluation of a monitoring system intervention: falls, injuries, and affect in nursing homes. *Clinical Nursing Research*, 16(4): 317–335.

Huang, H.L., Shyu, Y.L., Chen, M.C., Chen, S.T. and Lin, L.C. (2003) A pilot study on a home-based caregiver training program for improving caregiver self-efficacy and decreasing behavioral problems of elders with dementia in Taiwan. *International Journal of Geriatric Psychiatry*, 18: 337–345.

Iliffe, S., Wilcock, J. and Haworth, D. (2006) Obstacles to shared care for patients with dementia : a qualitative study. *Family Practice*, 23: 353–362.

Indigenous Allied Health Australia (2015) *Cultural Responsiveness In Action: An IAHA Framework*. Available at: http://iaha.com.au/wp-content/uploads/2015/08/2015-IAHA-Cultural-Responsiveness-Framework-WEB.pdf (accessed 14/09/16).

Inouye, S., Westendorp, R. and Saczynski, J. (2014) Delirium in elderly people. *Lancet*, 383: 911–922.

Institute for Health Improvement (2016) *How to Improve*. Available at: www.ihi.org/resources/Pages/HowtoImprove/default.aspx (accessed 10/09/16).

Jeon, Y.-H., Luscombe, G., Chenoweth, L., Stein-Parbury, J., Brodaty, H. and Haas, M. (2012) Staff Outcomes from the Caring for Aged Dementia Care REsident Study (CADRES): a cluster randomised trial. *International Journal of Nursing Studies*, 49: 508–518.

Jordan, M.E., Lanham, H.J., Crabtree, B.F., Nutting, P.A., Miller, W.L., Stange, K.C. and McDaniel, Jr., R.R. (2009) The role of conversation in healthcare interventions: enabling sensemaking and learning. *Implementation Science*, 4: 15.

Jordan, M., Lanham, H.J., Anderson, R.A. and McDaniel, R.R. (2010) Implications of complex adaptive systems theory for interpreting research about healthcare organizations. *Journal of Evaluation in Clinical Practice*, 16: 228–231.

Kerssens, C., Kumar, R., Adams, A., Knott, C., Matalenas, L., Sanford, J. and Rogers, W. (2015) Personalized technology to support older adults with and without cognitive impairment living at home. *American Journal of Alzheimer's Disease & Other Dementias*, 30(1): 85–97.

Kidd, C., Taggart, W. and Turkle, S. (2006) A sociable robot to encourage social interaction among the elderly. *In Proceedings 2006 IEEE International Conference on Robotics and Automation*. ICRA. pp.3972–3976.

Killett, A., Bowes, A., Brooker, D., Burns, D., Kelly, F., La Fontaine, J., Latham, I., O'Neill, M., Poland, F. and Wilson, M. (2013) What makes a real difference to resident experience? Digging deep into care home culture: the CHOICE (Care Home Organisations Implementing

Cultures of Excellence) research report. 025/0064. Available at: www.tsab.org.uk/wp-content/uploads/2015/11/CHOICE_final_report.pdf (accessed 21/01/16).

Killett, A., Burns, D., Kelly, F., Brooker, D., Bowes, A., LaFontaine, J., Latham, I., Wilson, M., and O'Nrill, M. (2016) Digging deep: how organisational culture affects care home residents' experiences. *Ageing and Society*, 36(1): 160–188.

Kitwood, T. (1997) *Dementia Reconsidered: The Person Comes First*. Buckingham: Open University Press.

Koren, M.J. (2010) Person-centered care for nursing home residents: the culture-change movement. *Health Affairs*, 29(2): 312–317.

Kotter, J. (2007) Leading change. Why transformation efforts fail. *Harvard Business Review. The tests of a leader*, January: 1–9.

Kotter, J. and Whitehead, L. (2010) *Buy-In: Saving Your Good Idea from Getting Shot Down*. Harvard Business Press Books.

Kotter International (2012) *Change Leadership*. Available at: www.kotterinternational.com/our-principles/change-leadership (accessed 17/07/14).

Landau, R., Auslander, G., Werner, S., Shoval, N. and Heinik, J. (2010) Families' and professional caregivers' views of using advanced technology to track people with dementia. *Qualitative Health Research*, 20(3): 409–419.

Leinenga, G. and Götz, J (2015) Scanning ultrasound removes amyloid-β and restores memory in an Alzheimer's disease mouse model. *Science Translational Medicine*, 7(278): 278ra33.

Libin, A. and Cohen-Mansfield, J. (2004) Therapeutic robocat for nursing home residents ith dementia: preliminary inquiry. *American Journal of Alzheimer's Disease and other Dementias*, 19(2): 111–116.

Liddle, J., Bennett, S., Allen, S., Lie, D.C., Standen, B. and Pachana, N.A. (2013) The stages of driving cessation for people with dementia: needs and challenges. *International Psychogeriatrics*, 25(12): 2033–2046.

Liddle, J., Reaston, T., Pachana, N., Mitchell, G. and Gustafsson, L. (2014) Is planning for driving cessation critical for the well-being and lifestyle of older drivers? *International Psychogeriatrics*, 26(7): 1111–1120.

Lin, C.-C., Lin, P.-Y., Lu, P.-K., Hsieh, G.-Y., Lee, W.-L. and Lee, R.-G. (2008) A healthcare integration system for disease assessment and safety monitoring of dementia patients. *Transactions on Information Technology in Biomedicine*, 12(5): 579–586.

Lindauer, A. and Harvath, T. (2015) The meanings caregivers ascribe to dementia-related changes in care recipients: a meta-ethnography. *Research in Gerontological Nursing*, 8(1): 39–48.

Lloyd, J., Patterson, T. and Muers, J. (2014) The positive aspects of caregiving in dementia: a critical review of the qualitative literature. *Dementia,* 16(6): 1534–61.

Logsdon, R.G., McCurry, S.M. and Teri, L. (2005) STAR-Caregivers: a community-based approach for teaching family caregivers to use behavioral strategies to reduce affective disturbances in persons with dementia. *Alzheimer's Care Quarterly*, 6: 146–153.

Lykens, K., Moayad, N., Biswas, S., Reyes-Ortiz, C. and Singh, K.P. (2014) Impact of a community based implementation of REACH II program for caregivers of Alzheimer's patients. *PLoS ONE*, 9(2): e89290.

Maas, M.L., Reed, D., Park, M., Specht, J.P., Schutte, D., Kelly, L.S., Swanson, E.A., Tripp-Reimer, T. and Buckwalter, K.C. (2004) Outcomes of family involvement in care intervention for caregivers of individuals with dementia. *Nursing Research*, 53(2): 76–86.

Maayan, N., Soares-Weiser, K. and Lee, H. (2014) Respite care for people with dementia and their carers. *Cochrane Database of Systematic Reviews*, Issue 1: Art. No. CD004396.

Magnusson, L., Sandman, L., Rosén, K.G. and Hanson, E. (2014) Extended safety and support systems for people with dementia living at home. *Journal of Assistive Technologies*, 8(4): 188–206.

Manley, K. and McCormack, B. (2004) Practice development: purpose, methodology, facilitation and evaluation. In B. McCormack, K. Manley and R. Garbett (eds), *Practice Development in Nursing*. Oxford: Blackwell Publishing. pp. 35–50.

Margot-Cattin, I. and Nygard, L. (2006) Access technology and dementia care: influences on residents' everyday lives in a secure unit. *Scandinavian Journal of Occupational Therapy*, 13: 113–124.

Mao, H.-F., Chang, L.-H, Yao, G., Chen, W.-Y. and Huang, W.-N. (2015) Indicators of perceived useful dementia care assistive technology: caregivers' perspectives. *Geriatrics Gerontology International*, 15: 1049–1057.

Marie Curie Cancer Care with Alzheimer's Society (2013) *Living and Dying with Dementia in England: Barriers to Care*. Available at: http://www2.mariecurie.org.uk/Documents/policy/dementia-report.pdf (accessed 22/08/16).

McCormack, B. (2011) Engaged scholarship and research impact: integrating the doing and using of research in practice. *Journal of Research in Nursing*, 16(2): 111–127.

McDaniel, R.R. and Driebe, D.J. (2001) Complexity science and health care management. In J.D. Blair, M.D. Fottler and G.T. Savage (eds), *Advances in Health Care Management. Vol. 2*. Stamford, CT: JAI Press. pp. 11–36.

Memon, M., Wagner, S., Pedersen, C., Hassan, F., Beevi, A. and Hansen, F. (2014) Ambient assisted living healthcare frameworks, platforms, standards, and quality attributes. *Sensors*, 14: 4312–4341.

Mental Capacity Act 2005. Available at: www.legislation.gov.uk/ukpga/2005/9/contents (accessed 10/03/17).

Millenaar, J.K., van Vliet, D., Bakker, C., Vernooij-Dassen, M.J.F.J., Koopmans, R.T.C.M., Verhey, F.R.J., de Vugt, M.E., Koopmans, R. and Rosness, T. (2014) The experiences and needs of children living with a parent with young onset dementia: results from the NeedYD study. *International Psychogeriatrics*, 26(12): 2001–2010.

Miller, S., Lepore, M., Lima, J., Shield, R. and Tyler, D. (2014a) Does the introduction of nursing home culture change practices and improve quality? *Journal of the American Geriatrics Society*, 62: 1675–1682.

Miller, S.C., Looze, J., Shield, R. et al. (2014b) Culture change practice in U.S. nursing homes: prevalence and variation by state Medicaid reimbursement policies. *Gerontologist*, 54: 434–445.

Mitchell, L., Burton, E. and Raman, S. (2004) Dementia friendly cities: designing intelligible neighbourhoods for life, *Journal of Urban Design*, 9(1): 89–101.

Mittelman, M.S., Epstein, C. and Pierzchala, A. (2003) *Counseling the Alzheimer's Caregiver: A Resource for Healthcare Professionals*. Chicago, Ill: AMA Press.

Mittelman, M.S., Roth, D.L., Coon, D.W. and Haley, W.E. (2004a) Sustained benefit of supportive intervention for depressive symptoms. *American Journal of Psychiatry*, 161: 850–856.

Mittelman, M.S., Roth, D.L., Haley, W.E. and Zarit, S.H. (2004b) Effects of a caregiver intervention on negative caregiver appraisals of behavior problems in patients with Alzheimer's disease: results of a randomized trial. *The Journals of Gerontology, Series B: Psychological Sciences & Social Sciences*, 59(1): 27–34.

Mittelman, M.S., Haley, W.E., Clay, O.J. and Roth, D.L. (2006) Improving caregiver well-being delays nursing home placement of patients with Alzheimer disease. *Neurology*, 67: 1592–1599.

Mittelman, M.S., Roth, D.L., Clay, O.J. and Haley, W.E. (2007) Preserving health of Alzheimer caregivers: impact of a spouse caregiver intervention. *American Journal of Geriatric Psychiatry*, 15(9): 780–789.

Miura, M., Ito, S., Takatsuka, R., Sugihara, T. and Kunifuji, S. (2009) An empirical study of an RFID mat sensor system in a group home. *Journal of Networks*, 4(2): 133–139.

Moye, J. and Marson, D.C. (2007) Assessment of decision-making capacity in older adults: an emerging area of practice and research. *Journals of Gerontology. Series B, Psychological Sciences and Social Sciences*, 62(1): 3–11.

Moyle, W., Olorenshaw, R., Wallis, M. and Borbasi, S. (2008) Best practice for the management of older people with dementia in the acute care setting: a review of the literature. *International Journal of Older People Nursing*, 3: 121–130.

Moyle, W., Borbasi, S., Walliss, M., Olorenshaw, R. and Gracia, N. (2011) Acute care management of older people with dementia: a qualitative perspective. *Journal of Clinical Nursing*, 20: 420–428.

Moyle, W., Cooke, M., Beattie, E., Jones, C., Klein, B., Cook, G. and Gray, C. (2013a) Exploring the effect of companion robots on emotions in older people with dementia: a pilot RCT. *Journal Gerontological Nursing*, 39: 46–53.

Moyle, W., Venturato, L., Cooke, M., Hughes, J., Van Wyk, S. and Marshall, J. (2013b) Promoting value in dementia care: staff, resident and family experience of the capabilities model of dementia care. *Aging and Mental Health*, 17(5): 587–594.

Moyle,W., Beattie, E., Draper, B., Shum, D., Lukman, T., Jones, C., O'Dwyer, S. and Mervin, C. (2015) Effect of an interactive therapeutic robotic animal on engagement, mood states, agitation and psychotropic drug use in people with dementia: a cluster-randomised controlled trial protocol. *BMJ Open*, 5.

Moyle, W., Venturato, L., Cooke, M., Murfield, J., Griffiths, S., Hughes, J. and Wolf, N. (2016) Evaluating the capabilities model of dementia care: a non-randomized controlled trial exploring resident quality of life and care staff attitudes and experiences. *International Psychogeriatric Association*, 1–10.

National Center for Health Statistics (2015) *Health, United States* With special feature on racial and ethnic health disparities. Hyattsville, MD. Available at: www.cdc.gov/nchs/data/hus/hus15.pdf#019 (accessed 01/09/2016).

National Collaborating Centre for Mental Health (2007) *Dementia: A NICE–SCIE Guideline on Supporting People with Dementia and their Carers in Health and Social Care*. National Clinical Practice Guideline Number 42. The British Psychological Society and Gaskell. Available at: www.scie.org.uk/publications/misc/dementia/dementia-fullguideline.pdf (accessed 27/11/16).

National LGBTI Health Alliance (2014) *Working Therapeutically with LGBTI Clients: A Practice Wisdom Resource*. Available at: www.lgbtihealth.org.au/sites/default/files/practice-wisdom-guide-online.pdf (accessed 14/09/16).

Nayton, K., Fielding, E., Brooks, D., Graham, F. and Beattie, E. (2014) Development of an education program to improve care of patients with dementia in an acute care setting. *The Journal of Continuing Education in Nursing*, 45(12): 552–8.

Neville, C., Beattie, E., Fielding, E. and MacAndrew, M. (2015) Literature review: use of respite by carers of people with dementia. *Health and Social Care in the Community*, 23: 51–63.

Nichols, L., Martindale-Adams, J., Burns, R., Graney, M.J. and Zuber, J. (2011) Translation of a dementia caregiver support program in a health care system – REACH VA. *Archives Internal Medicine*, 171(4): 353–359.

Niemeijer, A.R., Frederiks, B.J., Riphagen, I.I., Legemaate, J., Eefsting, J.A. and Hertogh, C.M. (2010) Ethical and practical concerns of surveillance technologies in residential care for people with dementia or intellectual disabilities: an overview of the literature. *International Psychogeriatrics*, 22(7): 1129–1142.

Nolan, L. (2006) Caring connections with older persons with dementia in an acute hospital setting: a hermeneutic interpretation of the staff nurse's experience. *International Journal of Older People Nursing*, 1: 208–215.

Nolan, M.R., Grant, G. and Keady, J. (1996) *Understanding Family Care*. Buckingham. Open University Press.

Nolan, M.R., Davies, S. and Grant, G. (eds) (2001) *Working with Older People and their Families*. Buckingham: Open University Press.

Nolan, M.R., Lundh, U., Grant, G. and Keady, J. (eds) (2003) *Partnerships in Family Care*. Maidenhead: Open University Press.

Nolan, M.R., Davies, S., et al. (2004) Beyond person-centred care: a new vision for gerontological nursing. *International Journal of Older People Nursing, in association with the Journal of Clinical Nursing*, 13(3a): 45–53.

Nolan, M.R., Brown, J. et al. (2006a) *The Senses Framework: Improving Care for Older People through a Relationship Centred Approach*. University of Sheffield. GRip Report.

Nolan, M., Davies, S. and Brown, J. (2006b) Transitions in care homes: towards relationship-centred care using the 'Senses Framework'. *Quality in Ageing*, 7(3): 5–15.

Nomura, Y. and Yamaji, K. (2008) Autonomous-type tracking robot with network environment. *Proceedings of 2008 IEEE International Conference on Mechatronics and Automation*. 168–173.

Olazarán, J., Reisberg, B., Clare, L. et al. (2010) Nonpharmacological therapies in Alzheimer's disease: a systematic review of efficacy. *Dementia and Geriatric Cognitive Disorders*, 30: 161–178.

Olsson, A., Engström, M., Asenlof, P., Skovdahl, K. and Lampic, C. (2015) Effects of tracking technology on daily life of persons with dementia: three experimental single-case studies. *American Journal of Alzheimer's Disease & Other Dementias*, 30(1): 29–40.

Olsson, A., Engström, M., Skovdahl, K., and Lampic, C. (2012) My, your and our needs for safety and security: relatives' reflections on using information and communication technology in dementia care. *Scandinavian Journal Caring Science*, 26: 104–112.

Orpwood, R., Chadd, J., Howcroft, D., Sixsmith, A., Torrington, J., Gibson, G. and Chalfont, G. (2010) Designing technology to improve quality of life for people with dementia: user-led approaches. *Universal Access in the Information Society*, 9(3): 249–259.

Owen, T. (2006) *My Home Life: Quality of Life in Care homes*. Help the Aged. Available at: http://myhomelife.org.uk/wp-content/uploads/2014/11/mhl_report.pdf (accessed 21/01/16).

Parker, D., Mills, S. and Abbey, R.N.J. (2008) Effectiveness of interventions that assist caregivers to support people with dementia living in the community: a systematic review. *International Journal of Evidence Based Healthcare*, 6: 137–172.

Pearlin, L.I., Mullin, J.T., Semple, S.J. and Skaff, M.M. (1990) Caregiving and the stress process: an overview of concepts and their measures. *The Gerontologist*, 30(5): 583–594.

Petriwskyj, A., Parker, D., Brown Wilson, C., and Gibson, A. (2016a) What health and aged care culture change models mean for residents and their families: a systematic review. *The Gerontologist*, 56(2): e12–20.

Petriwskyj, A., Parker, D., Brown Wilson, C. and Gibson, A. (2016b) Evaluation of subscription-based culture change models in care settings: findings from a systematic review. *The Gerontologist*, 56(2): 12–20.

Pinquart, M. and Sorensen, S. (2003) Predictors of caregiver burden and depressive mood: a meta-analysis. *Journal of Gerontology, Psychological Sciences*, 58: 112–128.

Pinquart, M. and Sorensen, S. (2004) Associations of caregivers' stressors and uplifts with subjective well-being and depressive mood: a meta-analytic comparison. *Aging & Mental Health*, 8(5): 438–449.

Pinquart, M. and Sorensen, S. (2005) Ethnic differences in stressors, resources, and psychological outcomes of family caregiving: a meta-analysis. *The Gerontologist*, 45(1): 90–106.

Pinquart, M. and Sorensen, S. (2006a) Helping caregivers of persons with dementia: which interventions work and how large are their effects? *International Psychogeriatrics*: 1–19.

Pinquart, M. and Sorensen, S. (2006b) Gender differences in caregiver stressors, social resources, and health: an updated meta-analysis. *Journal of Gerontology: Psychological Sciences*, 61B(1): 33–45.

Pinquart, M. and Sorensen, S. (2011) Spouses, adult children, and children-in-law as carers of older adults: a meta-analytic comparison. *Psychology of Aging*, 26(1): 1–14.

Plsek, P. and Greenhalgh, T. (2001) Complexity science: the challenge of complexity in health care. *British Medical Journal*, 323: 625–8.

Plsek, P. (2003) Complexity and the adoption of innovation in health care: accelerating quality improvement in health care strategies to speed the diffusion of evidence-based innovations, Conference held in Washington, D.C. January 27–28. Available at www.nihcm.org/pdf/Plsek.pdf (accessed 23/11/16).

Pol, P., van Nes, F., van Hartingsveldt, M., Buurman, B., de Rooij, S. and Kröse, B. (2016) Older people's perspectives regarding the use of sensor monitoring in their home. *Gerontologist*, 56(3): 485–493.

Popescu, M. and Mahnot, A. (2012) Early illness recognition in older adults using in-home monitoring sensors and multiple instance learning. *Methods of Informatics in Medicine*, 51(4): 359–367.

Porock, D., Clissett, P., Harwood, R.H. and Gladman, J. (2015) Disruption, control and coping: responses of and to the person with dementia in hospital. *Ageing & Society*, 35(1): 37–63.

Prensky, M. (2001) Digital natives, digital immigrants. *On the Horizon*, 9(5): 1–6.

Prince, M., Bryce, R. and Ferri, C. (2011) *Alzheimer's Disease International – World Alzheimer Report 2011: The Benefits of Early Diagnosis and Intervention*. Available at: www.alz.co.uk/research/WorldAlzheimerReport2011.pdf (accessed 08/01/16).

Prince, M., Knapp, M., Guerchet, M., McCrone, P., Prina, M., Comas-Herrera, A., Wittenberg, R., Adelaja, B., Hu, B., King, D., Rehill, A. and Salimkumar, D. (2014) *Dementia UK* (second edition). Alzheimer's Society.

Prince, M., Wimo, A., Guerchet, M., Ali, G.C., Wu, Y.-T. and Prina, M. (2015) *World Alzheimers Report 2015: Global Impact of Dementia. An Analysis of Prevalence, Incidence, Costs and Trends*. Alzheimer's Disease International (ADI), London. Available at: www.worldalzreport2015.org/downloads/world-alzheimer-report-2015.pdf (accessed 10/01/16).

Rantz, M.J., Dorman-Marek, K., Aud, M., Johnson, R.A., Otto, D. and Porter, R. (2005) TigerPlace: a new future for older adults. *Journal of Nursing Care Quality*, 20: 1–4.

Rantz, M.J., Skubic, M., Koopman, R., Phillips, L., Alexander, G., Miller, S. and Guevara, R. (2011) Using sensor networks to detect urinary tract infections in older adults. *Proceedings of the 13th IEEE International Conference on E-Health Networking and Applications*. PID1858641.

Rantz, M.J., Skubic, M., Koopman, R.J., Alexander, G., Phillips, L., Musterman, K.I., Back, J.R., Aud, M.A., Galambos, C., Guevara, R.D. and Miller, S.J. (2012) Automated technology to speed recognition of signs of illness in older adults. *Journal of Gerontological Nursing*, 38(4): 18–23.

Rantz, M.J., Skubic, M., Miller, S., Galambos, C., Alexander, G.L., Keller, J. and Popescu, M. (2013a) Sensor technology to support aging in place. *Journal of the American Medical Directors Association*, 14: 386–391.

Rantz, M.J., Zwygart-Stauffacher, M., Flesner, M. et al. (2013b) The influence of teams to sustain quality improvement in nursing homes that 'need improvement'. *Journal of the American Medical Directors Association*, 14(1): 48–52.

Rantz, M., Skubic, M., Popescu, M., Galambos, C., Koopman, R.J., Alexander, G.L., Phillips, L.J., Musterman, K., Back, J. and Miller, S.J. (2015a) A new paradigm of technology-enabled 'vital signs' for early detection of health change for older adults. *Gerontology*, 61(3): 281–290.

Rantz, M., Lane, K., Phillips, L.J., Despins, L.A., Galambos, C., Alexander, G.L., Koopman, R.J., Hicks, L., Skubic, M. and Miller, S.J. (2015b) Enhanced RN care coordination with sensor technology: impact on length of stay and cost in aging in place housing. *Nursing Outlook*, 63: 650–655.

Raymond, M., Warner, A., Davies N., Baishnab, E., Manthorpe, J. and Iliffe, S. (2014a) Evaluating educational initiatives to improve palliative care for people with dementia: a narrative review. *Dementia*, 13(3): 366–381.

Raymond, M., Warner, A., Davies, N., Iliffe, S., Manthorpe, J. and Ahmedzhai, S. (2014b) Palliative care services for people with dementia: a synthesis of the literature reporting the views and experiences of professionals and family carers. *Dementia*, 13(1): 96–110.

Reed, J. and Card, A. (2016) The problem with Plan-Do-Study-Act Cycles. *BMJ Quality Safety*, 25: 147–152.

Reilly, S., Miranda-Castillo, C., Malouf, R., Hoe, J., Toot, S., Challis, D. and Orrell, M. (2015) Case management approaches to home support for people with dementia. *Cochrane Database of Systematic Reviews*, 1: Art. No. CD008345.

Roberts, G., Morley, C., Walters, W., Malta, S. and Doyle, C. (2015) Caring for people with dementia in residential aged care: successes with a composite person-centered care model featuring Montessori-based activities. *Geriatric Nursing*, 36(2): 106–110.

Robinson, L., Hutchings, D., Corner, L., Finch,T., Hughes, J., Brittain, K. and Bond, J. (2007) Balancing rights and risks: conflicting perspectives in the management of wandering in dementia. *Health, Risk & Society*, 9(4): 389–406.

Robinson, L., Dickinson, C., Rousseau, N., Beyer, F., Clark, A., Hughes, J., Howel, D. and Exley, C. (2012) A systematic review of the effectiveness of advance care planning interventions for people with cognitive impairment and dementia. *Age and Ageing*, 41: 263–269.

Rokstad, A., Røsvik, J., Kirkevold, O., Selbaek, G., Benth, J. and Engedal, K. (2013) The effect of person-centred dementia care to prevent agitation and other neuropsychiatric symptoms and enhance quality of life in nursing home patients: a 10-month randomized controlled trial. *Dementia and Geriatric Cognitive Disorders*, 36: 340–353.

Rossor, M.N., Fox, N.C., Mummery, C.J., Schott, J.M. and Warren, J.D. (2010) The diagnosis of young-onset dementia. *Lancet Neurology*, 9: 793–806.

Rosvik, J., Kirkevold, M., Engedal, K., Brooker, D. and Kirkevold, O. (2011) A model for using the VIPS framework for person-centred care for persons with dementia in nursing homes: a qualitative evaluative study. *International Journal of Older People Nursing*, 6: 227–236.

Rosvik, J., Broker, D., Mjorud, M. and Kirkevold, O. (2013) What is person-centred care in dementia? Clinical review into practice: the development of the VIPS practice model. *Reviews in Clinical Gerontology*, 23: 155–163.

Roth, D., Mittelman, M., Clay, O., Madan, A. and Haley, W. (2005) Changes in social support as mediators of the impact of a psychosocial intervention for spouse caregivers of persons with Alzheimer's disease. *Psychology and Aging*, 20(4): 634–644.

Rouse, K. (2008) Health care as a complex adaptive system: implications for design and management. *The Bridge*, 38(1): 17–25.

Royal College of Psychiatrists (2013) *National Audit of Dementia Care in General Hospitals 2012–13: Second Round Audit Report and Update*. Editors: J. Young, C. Hood, A. Gandesha and R. Souza. London: HQIP. Available at: www.rcpsych.ac.uk/pdf/NAD%20 NATIONAL%20REPORT%202013%20reports%20page.pdf (accessed 30/08/16).

Ryan, T., Nolan, M., Reid, D. and Enderby, P. (2008) Using the senses framework to achieve relationship-centred dementia care services: a case example. *Dementia: The International Journal of Social Research and Practice*, 7(1):71–93.

Rycroft-Malone, J. (2004) The PARIHS framework – a framework for guiding the implementation of evidence-based practice. *Journal of Nursing Care Quality*, 19(4): 297–304.

Samsi, K. and Manthorpe, J. (2011) 'I live for today': a qualitative study investigating older people's attitudes to advance planning. *Health and Social Care in the Community*, 19(1): 52–59.

Samsi, K. and Manthorpe, J. (2013) Everyday decision-making in dementia: findings from a longitudinal interview study of people with dementia and family carers. *International Psychogeriatrics*, 25(6): 949–961.

Savenstedt, S., Sandma, P. and Zingmark, K. (2006) The duality in using information and communication technology in elder care. *Journal of Advanced Nursing*, 56(1): 17–25.

Schein, E. (2010) *Organisational Culture and Leadership* (fourth edition). California: Josey Bass.

Schikhof, Y. and Mulder, I. (2008) Under watch and ward at night: design and evaluation of a remote monitoring system for dementia care. Symposium of the Austrian HCI and Usability Engineering Group USAB 2008: HCI and Usability for Education and Work. pp. 475–486, Volume 5298 of the book series Lecture Notes in Computer Science (LNCS).

Schikhof, Y., Mulder, I. and Choenni, S. (2010) Who will watch(over)me? Humane monitoring in dementia care. *International Journal of Human–Computer Studies*, 68: 410–422.

Schneidert, M., Hurst, R., Miller, J. and Bedirhan Ustun, T. (2003) The role of environment in the international classification of functioning. *Disability and Health (ICF) Disability and Rehabilitation*, 25(11–12): 588–595.

Schoenmakers, B., Buntinx, F. and Delepeleire, J. (2010) Supporting the dementia family caregiver: the effect of home care intervention on general well-being. *Aging and Mental Health*, 14(1): 44–56.

Schulz, R., Burgio, L., Burns, R., Eisdorfer, C. and Gallagher-Thompson, D. (2003) Resources for enhancing Alzheimer's caregiver health (REACH): overview, site-specific outcomes, and future directions. *The Gerontologist*, 43(4): 514–520.

Scott, T., Mannion, R., Davies, H. and Marshall, M. (2003) Implementing culture change in health care: theory and practice. *International Journal for Quality in Health Care*, 15(2): 111–118.

Scott, T., Mittelman, M., Beattie, E., Parker, D. and Neville, C. (2015) Translating training in the NYU Caregiver Intervention in Australia: maintaining fidelity and meeting graduate standards in an online continuing professional education setting. *Educational Gerontology*, 41(10): 710–722.

Sellgren, S.F., Ekvall, G. and Tomson, G. (2008) Leadership behaviour of nurse managers in relation to job satisfaction and work climate. *Journal of Nursing Management*, 16: 578–587.

Semiatin, A. and O'Connor, M. (2012) The relationship between self-efficacy and positive aspects of caregiving in Alzheimer's disease caregivers. *Aging & Mental Health*, 16(6): 683–688.

Setterlund, D., Tilse, C. and Wilson, J. (2002) Older people and substitute decision making legislation: limits to informed choice. *Australasian Journal on Ageing*, 21(3): 128–133.

Sheard, D. (2014) Achieving culture change: a whole organisation approach. *Nursing and Residential Care*, 16(6): 329–332.

Siddiqi, N., Harrison, J.K., Clegg, A., Teale, E.A., Young, J., Taylor, J. and Simpkins, S.A. (2016) Interventions for preventing delirium in hospitalised non-ICU patients. *Cochrane Database of Systematic Reviews 2016*, Issue 3: Art. No. CD005563.

Simpson, P., Horne, M., Brown, L.E.J., Brown Wilson, C., Dickinson, T. and Torkington, K. (2015) 'We've had our sex life way back': older care home residents in Northwest England

and sexuality, intimacy and erotophobia. *Ageing and Society,* doi: http://dx.doi.org/10.1017/S0144686X15001105.

Simpson, P., Brown Wilson, C., Horne, M., Brown, L.E.J. and Dickinson, T. (2016) The challenges and opportunities in researching intimacy and sexuality in care homes accommodating older people: a feasibility study. *Journal of Advanced Nursing*, doi: 10.1111/jan.13080.

Smith, M., Gerdner, L., Hall, G. and Buckwalter, K. (2004) History, development, and future of the progressively lowered stress threshold: a conceptual model for dementia care. *Journal of the American Geriatrics Society*, 52: 1755–1760.

Snowden, D. and Boone, M. (2007) A leaders' framework for decision making. *Harvard Business Review*, November: 69–76.

Snowdon, D. (1997) Aging and Alzheimer's Disease: lessons from the Nun Study. *Gerontologist*, 37(2): 150–156.

Soderstrom, I.M., Benzein, E. and Saveman, B.I. (2003) Nurses' experiences of interactions with family members in intensive care units. *Scandinavian Journal of Caring Sciences*, 17(2): 185–192.

Sorensen, S. and Pinquart, M. (2005) Racial and ethnic differences in the relationship of caregiving stressors, resources, and sociodemographic variables to caregiver depression and perceived physical health. *Aging & Mental Health*, 9(5): 482–495.

Stroebel, C., McDaniel, Jr., R., Crabtree, B.F., Miller, W.L., Nutting, P.A. and Stange, K.C. (2005) Using complexity science to inform a reflective practice improvement process. *Joint Commission Journal on Quality and Safety*, 31: 438–46.

Subramaniam, P., Woods, B. and Whitaker, C. (2014) Life review and life story books for people with mild to moderate dementia: a randomised controlled trial. *Aging & Mental Health*, 18(3): 363–375.

Sugihara, T. and Fujinami, T. (2011) Emerging triage support environment for dementia care with camera system. International Conference on Ergonomics and Health Aspects of Work with Computers, *Lecture Notes in Computer Science (LNCS),* 6779: 149–158.

Sugihara, T., Nakagawa, K., Fujinami, T. and Takatsuka, R. (2008) Evaluation of a prototype of the mimamori-care system for persons with dementia. 12th International Conference on Knowledge-Based Intelligent Information and Engineering Systems, *Knowledge-Based Intelligent Information and Engineering Systems* 2008, Part II, LNAI 5178: 839–846.

Surr, C.A. (2006) Preservation of self in people with dementia living in residential care: a socio-biographical approach. *Social Science and Medicine*, 62: 1720–1730.

Takatsuka, R. and Fujinami, T. (2005) Aware group home: person-centered care as creative problem solving knowledge-based intelligent information and engineering systems. 9th International Conference. *Lecture Notes in Computer Science (LNCS)*, 3684: 451–457.

Taylor, M.J., McNicholas, C., Nicolay, C., Darzi, A., Bell, D. and Reed, J. (2013) Systematic review of the application of the plan–do–study–act method to improve quality in healthcare. *BMJ Quality and Safety*, 0: 1–9.

Teri, L., Logsdon, R.G., Uomoto, J. and McCurry, S. (1997) Behavioral treatment of depression in dementia patients: a controlled clinical trial. *Journal of Gerontology Series B: Psychological Sciences*, 52: 159–166.

Teri, L., Gibbons, L.E., McCurry, S.M., Logsdon, R.G., Buchner, D.M., Barlow, W.E. and Larson, E.B. (2003) Exercise plus behavioral management in patients with Alzheimer disease: a randomized controlled trial. *Journal of the American Medical Association*, 290: 2015–2022.

Teri, L., McCurry, S.M., Logsdon, R.G. and Gibbons, L.E. (2005) Training community consultants to help family members improve dementia care: a randomized controlled trial. *The Gerontologist*, 45: 802–811.

Teri, L., McKenzie, G., Logsdon, R., McCurry, S., Bollin, S., Mead, J. and Menne, H. (2012) Translation of two evidence-based programs for training families to improve care of persons with dementia. *Gerontologist*, 52(4): 452–459.

Thompson, C., Spilsbury, K., Hall, J., Birks, Y., Barnes, C. and Adamson, J. (2007) Systematic review of information and support interventions for caregivers of people with dementia. *BMC Geriatrics*, 7(18): 1–12.

Tilse, C., Setterlund, D., Wilson, J. and Rosenman, L. (2005) Minding the money: a growing responsibility for informal carers. *Ageing and Society*, 25(2): 215–227.

Todd, S., Barr, S. and Passmore, A.P. (2013) Cause of death in Alzheimer's disease: a cohort study. *QJM: An International Journal of Medicine*, 106(8): 747–53.

Travers, C., Byrne, G., Pachana, N., Klein, K. and Gray, L. (2012) Prospective observational study of dementia and delirium in the acute hospital setting. *Internal Medicine Journal*, 43: 262–269.

Travers, C., Beattie, E., Martin-Khan, M. and Fielding, E. (2013) A survey of the Queensland healthcare workforce: attitudes towards dementia care and training. *BMC Geriatrics*, 13: 101.

Tresolini C.P. and the Pew-Fetzer Task Force (1994) *Health Professions Education and Relationship-Centred Care*. San Francisco, CA: Pew Health Professions Commission.

Tuszynski, Mh., Yang, Jh., Barba, D., Hoi-Sang, U., Bakay, R., Pay, M.M., Masliah, E., Conner, Jm., Kobalka, P., Roy, S. and Nagahara, A.H. (2015) Nerve growth factor gene therapy: activation of neuronal responses in Alzheimer Disease. *JAMA Neurology*, 72(10): 1139–1147.

Utley-Smith, Q., Colón-Emeric, C., Lekan-Rutledge, D., Ammarell, N., Bailey, D., Corazzini, K., Piven, M. and Anderson, R.A. (2009) The nature of staff – family interactions in nursing homes: staff perceptions. *Journal of Aging Studies*, 23(3): 168–177.

van der Steen, J., Radbruch, L., Hertogh, C., de Boer, M., Hughes, J., Larkin, P., Francke, A., Jünger, S., Gove, D., Firth, P., Koopmans, R. and Volicer, L. on behalf of the European Association for Palliative Care (EAPC) (2014) White paper defining optimal palliative care in older people with dementia: a Delphi study and recommendations from the European Association for Palliative Care. *Palliative Medicine*, 28(3): 197–209.

van Hoof, J., Kort, H., van Waarde, H. and Blom, M.M. (2007) Environmental interventions and the design of homes for older adults with dementia: an overview. *American Journal of Alzheimers Disease and Other Dementias*, 25: 202.

van Vliet, D., de Vugt, M.E., Bakker, C., Koopmans, R.T. and Verhey, F.R. (2010) Impact of early onset dementia on caregivers: a review. *International Journal of Geriatric Psychiatry*, 25(11): 1091–100.

van Vliet, D., de Vugt, M.E., Bakker, C., Pijnenburg, Y.A., Vernooij-Dassen, M.J., Koopmans, R.T. et al. (2013) Time to diagnosis in young-onset dementia as compared with late-onset dementia. *Psychological Medicine*, 43(2): 423–432.

Volicer, L. and Hurley, A.C. (2003) Management of behavioral symptoms in progressive degenerative dementias. *Journal of Gerontology: Medical Sciences*, 58A(9): 837–845.

Wada, K. and Shibata, T. (2007) Social effects of robot therapy in a care house: change of social network of the residents for two months. In *International Conference on Robotics and Automation*. pp. 1250–1255. IEEE.

Wada, K., Shibata, T., Saito, T. and Tanie, K. (2004) Effects of robot assisted activity for elderly people and nurses at a day service center. *Proceedings of the IEEE*, 92(11): 1780–1788.

Wada, K., Shibata, T., Musha, T. and Kimura, S. (2008) Robot therapy for elders affected by dementia. *IEEE Engineering Medicine and Biology*, 27(4): 53–60.

Wada, K., Shibata, T. and Kawaguchi, Y. (2009) Long-term robot therapy in a health service facility for the aged: a case study for 5 years. IEEE International Conference on Rehabilitation Robotics, June 2009, pp. 930–933.

Waller, S., Masterson, A. and Finn, H. (2013) Improving the patient experience: developing supportive design for people with dementia. The King's Fund's Enhancing the Healing Environment Programme 2009–2012. London: The King's Fund. London. Available at: www.kingsfund.org.uk/sites/files/kf/field/field_publication_file/developing-supportive-design-for-people-with-dementia-kingsfund-jan13_0.pdf (accessed 30/06/16).

Want, R. (2006) An introduction to RFID technology. *IEEE Pervasive Computing*, 5(1): 25–33.

Wigg J.M. (2010) Liberating the wanderers: using technology to unlock doors for those living with dementia. *Sociology of Health & Illness*, 32(2): 288–303.

Wimo, A. and Prince, M. (2010) *World Alzheimer Report 2010: The Global Economic Impact of Dementia*. London, Alzheimer's Disease International.

World Health Organisation (2015) First WHO ministerial conference on global action against dementia: meeting report, WHO Headquarters, Geneva, Switzerland, 16–17 March 2015. Available at: www.who.int/mental_health/neurology/dementia/ministerial_conference_2015_report/en/ (accessed 10/01/16).

Zwijsen, S., Alistair, R., Niemeijer, A., Cees, M.P.M. and Hertogh, C. (2011) Ethics of using assistive technology in the care for community-dwelling elderly people: an overview of the literature. *Aging & Mental Health*, 15(4): 419–427.

Zwijsen, S.A., Depla, M., Francke, A., Niemeijer, A. and Hertogh, C. (2012) Surveillance technology: an alternative to physical restraints? A qualitative study among professionals working in nursing homes for people with dementia. *International Journal of Nursing Studies*, 49: 212–219.

Index